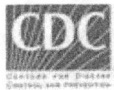

(Released 06/2013)

I0425919

Health Insurance Coverage: Early Release of Estimates From the National Health Interview Survey, 2012

by Robin A. Cohen, Ph.D., and Michael E. Martinez, M.P.H., M.H.S.A.
Division of Health Interview Statistics, National Center for Health Statistics

Highlights

- In 2012, 45.5 million persons of all ages (14.7%) were uninsured at the time of interview, 57.7 million (18.6%) had been uninsured for at least part of the year prior to interview, and 34.1 million (11.1%) had been uninsured for more than a year at the time of interview.
- In 2012, 4.9 million (6.6%) children under age 18 were uninsured at the time of interview.
- Among adults aged 19–25, the percentage uninsured at the time of interview was 26.4% (7.9 million) in 2012.
- In 2012, the percentage of persons who were uninsured at the time of interview, among the 43 states included in this report, ranged from 4.8% in Massachusetts to 20.9% in Oklahoma, South Carolina, and Texas.
- In 2012, 31.1% of persons under age 65 with private health insurance at the time of interview were enrolled in a high-deductible health plan (HDHP), including 10.8% who were enrolled in a consumer-directed health plan (CDHP). More than 50% of persons with a private plan obtained by means other than through employment were enrolled in an HDHP.
- An estimated 21.6% of persons with private health insurance were in a family with a flexible spending account (FSA) for medical expenses.

Introduction

The Centers for Disease Control and Prevention's (CDC) National Center for Health Statistics (NCHS) is releasing selected estimates of health insurance coverage for the civilian noninstitutionalized U.S. population based on data from the 2012 National Health Interview Survey (NHIS), along with comparable estimates from the 1997–2011 NHIS. Data analyses for the 2012 NHIS were based on 108,131 persons in the Family Core.

Three measures of lack of health insurance coverage are provided: (a) uninsured at the time of interview, (b) uninsured at least part of the year prior to interview (which also includes persons uninsured for more than a year), and (c) uninsured for more than a year at the time of interview. Estimates of public and private coverage are also presented.

This report includes estimates for adults aged 19–25 (Tables 1, 2, 3, 7–11), which are of special interest because of provisions of the Affordable Care Act of 2010 (P.L. 111–148, P.L. 111–152) (ACA). Under ACA, since September 23, 2010, young adults aged 19–25 can be covered under their parent's employer-sponsored or individually purchased health insurance. Tables 8–11 present quarterly estimates for adults aged 19–25. Table 8 also provides quarterly estimates for adults aged 26–35, for comparison.

For individuals with private health insurance, estimates are presented in Tables 12 and 13 for enrollment in high-deductible health plans (HDHPs), enrollment in consumer-directed health plans (CDHPs), and being in a family with a flexible spending account (FSA) for medical expenses.

State-level estimates of uninsured at the time of interview and public and private coverage are presented in Table 14.

This report is updated quarterly and is part of the NHIS Early Release (ER) Program, which releases updated

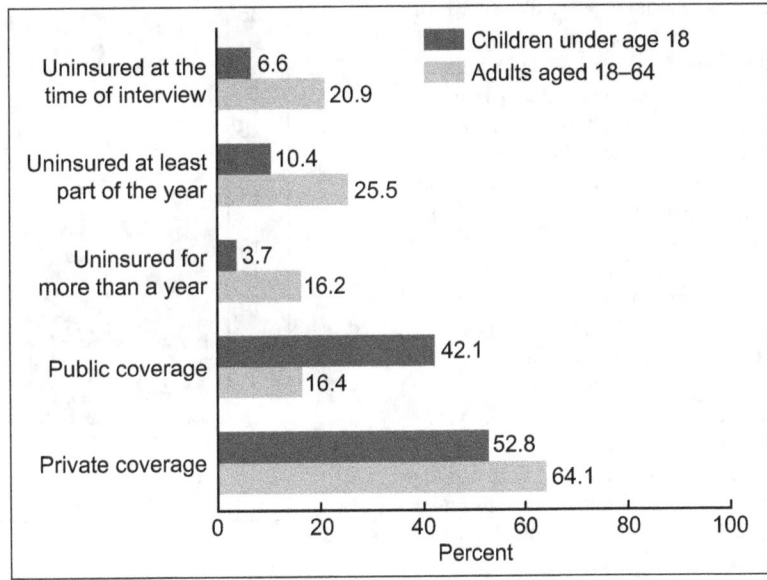

Figure 1. Percentage of persons without health insurance, by three measurements and age group, and percentage of persons with health insurance at the time of interview, by coverage type and age group: United States, 2012

NOTE: Data are based on household interviews of a sample of the civilian noninstitutionalized population.

DATA SOURCE: CDC/NCHS, National Health Interview Survey, 2012, Family Core component.

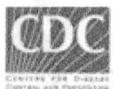

selected estimates that are available from the NHIS website at: http://www.cdc.gov/nchs/nhis.htm.

For more information about NHIS and the ER Program, see the **Technical Notes** and **Additional Early Release Program Products** sections at the end of this report.

Results

Lack of health insurance coverage

In 2012, the percentage of persons uninsured at the time of interview was 14.7% (45.5 million) for persons of all ages, 16.9% (45.2 million) for persons under age 65, 20.9% (40.3 million) for persons aged 18–64, and 6.6% (4.9 million) for children under age 18 (**Tables 1** and **2**). Among adults aged 19–25, 26.4% (7.9 million) lacked coverage at the time of interview in 2012. For all age groups, there were no significant changes between 2011 and 2012 in the percentage of persons uninsured at the time of interview.

Based on data from the 2012 NHIS, a total of 57.7 million (18.6%) persons of all ages were uninsured for at least part of the year prior to interview (**Tables 1** and **2**). Adults aged 18–64 were more than twice as likely (25.5%) as children (10.4%) to experience this lack of coverage. Among adults aged 19–25, 33.0% had been uninsured for at least part of the past year in 2012, a decrease from 2011 (36.1%). However, among the other age groups presented in **Table 1**, there were no significant changes between 2011 and 2012 in the percentage of persons who were uninsured for at least part of the year prior to interview.

Data from 2012 also revealed that 12.7% (33.9 million) of persons under age 65 (16.2% of adults and 3.7% of children) had been uninsured for more than a year (**Tables 1** and **2**). Adults aged 18–64 were more than four times as likely as children to have been uninsured for more than a year (**Figure 1**). Among adults aged 19–25, the percentage uninsured for more than a year was 19.6% (**Table 1**). For all age groups, there were no significant

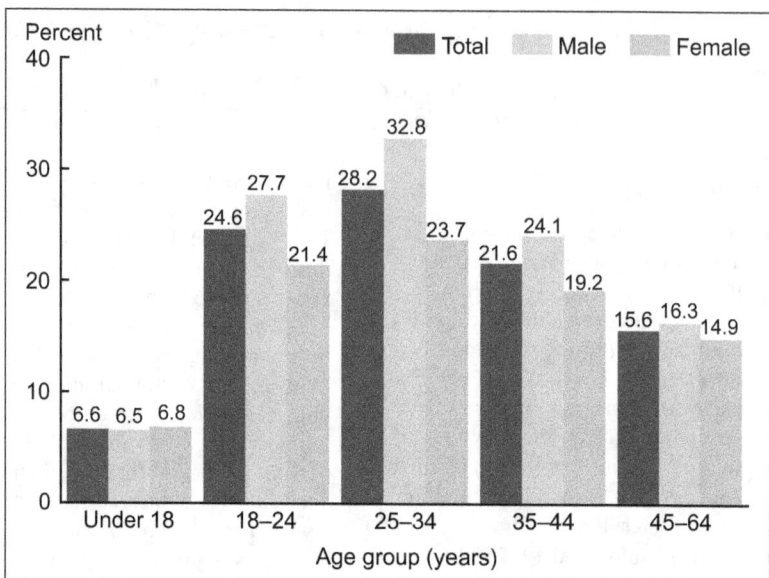

Figure 2. Percentage of persons under age 65 without health insurance coverage at the time of interview, by age group and sex: United States, 2012

NOTE: Data are based on household interviews of a sample of the civilian noninstitutionalized population.

DATA SOURCE: CDC/NCHS, National Health Interview Survey, 2012, Family Core component.

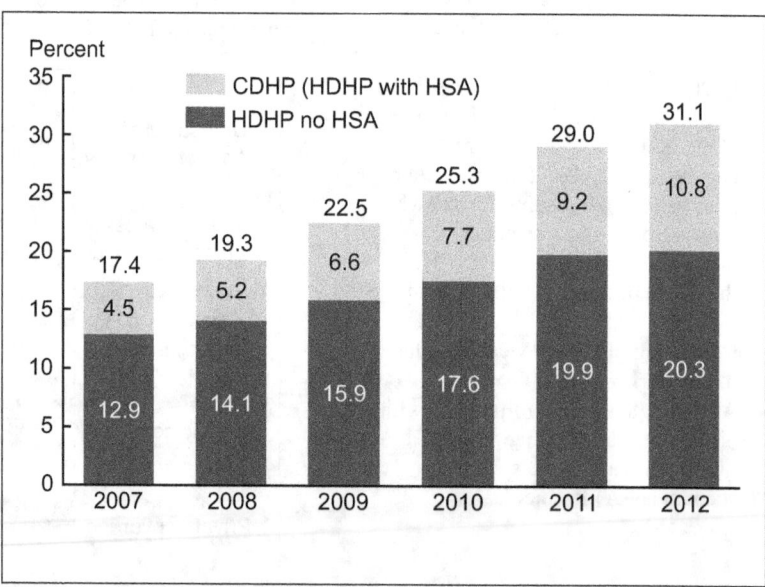

Figure 3. Percentages of persons under age 65 who are enrolled in a high-deductible health plan without a health savings account, or in a consumer-directed health plan, among those with private health insurance: United States, 2007–2012

NOTES: CDHP is consumer-directed health plan, which is a high-deductible health plan (HDHP) with a health savings account (HSA). HDHP no HSA is a high-deductible health plan without an HSA. The individual components of HDHPs may not add up to the total, due to rounding. Data are based on household interviews of a sample of the civilian noninstitutionalized population.

DATA SOURCE: CDC/NCHS, National Health Interview Survey, 2007–2012, Family Core component.

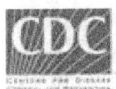

changes between 2011 and 2012 in the percentage of persons who had been uninsured for more than a year.

Public and private coverage

In 2012, 23.5% of persons under age 65 were covered by public health plans at the time of interview (Table 3). More than two-fifths of children (42.1%) were covered by a public plan, compared with 16.4% of adults aged 18–64 (Figure 1). Public coverage among adults aged 19–25 was 17.5% (Table 3). For all age groups, there were no significant changes in public coverage between 2011 and 2012.

In 2012, 61.0% of persons under age 65 were covered by private health insurance plans at the time of interview (Table 3). Slightly less than two-thirds (64.1%) of adults aged 18–64 were covered by a private plan, compared with 52.8% of children under age 18 (Figure 1). Among adults aged 19–25, 57.2% were covered by a private plan. For all age groups, there were no significant changes in private coverage between 2011 and 2012.

Insurance coverage, by poverty status

In 2012, 7.5% of poor children, 10.1% of near-poor children, and 4.5% of not-poor children (see Technical Notes for definition of poverty status) did not have health insurance coverage at the time of interview (Table 4). During the same period, 40.1% of poor, 39.2% of near-poor, and 11.4% of not-poor adults aged 18–64 lacked coverage at the time of interview.

In 2012, 85.9% of poor children, 61.0% of near-poor children, and 15.2% of not-poor children were covered by a public health plan at the time of interview (Table 5). In addition, for the age group 18–64, 40.8% of poor adults, 25.2% of near-poor adults, and 8.7% of not-poor adults were covered by a public plan.

In 2012, 8.8% of poor children, 31.1% of near-poor children, and 81.3% of not-poor children were covered by private health insurance at the time of interview (Table 6). In

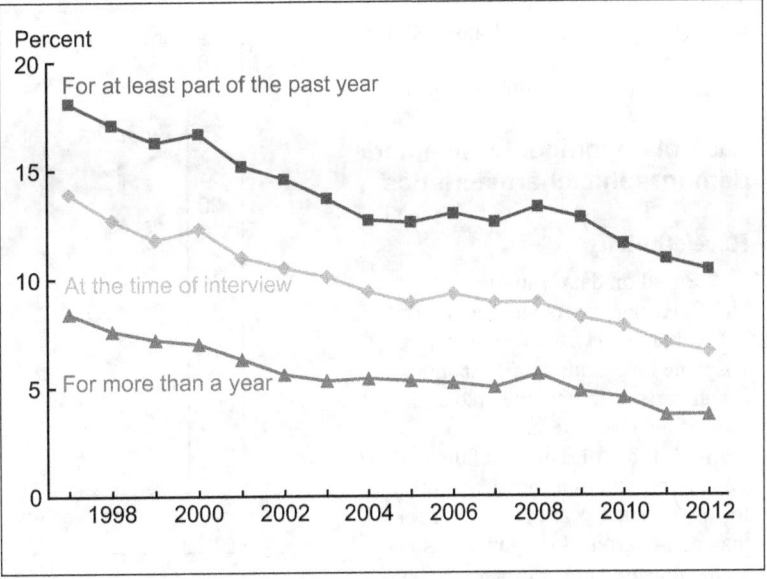

Figure 4. Percentages of children under age 18 who lacked health insurance coverage at the time of interview, for at least part of the past year, or for more than a year: United States, 1997–2012

NOTE: Data are based on household interviews of a sample of the civilian noninstitutionalized population.

DATA SOURCE: CDC/NCHS, National Health Interview Survey, 1997–2012, Family Core component.

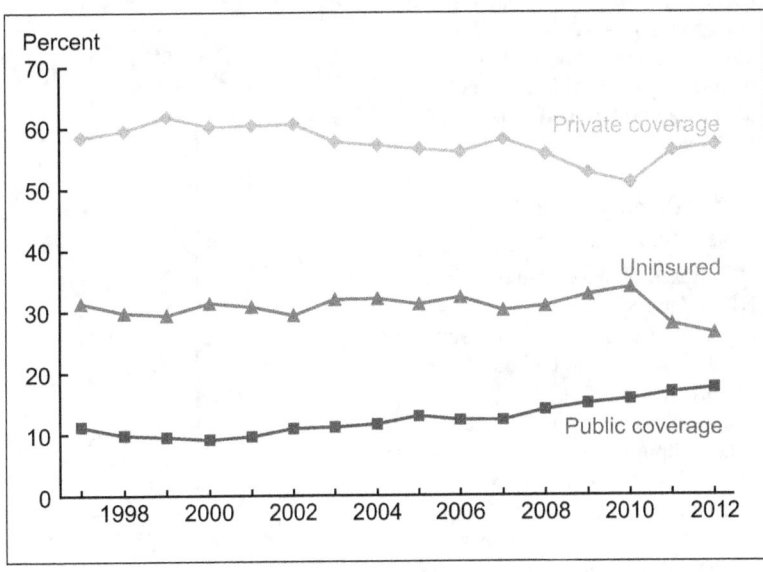

Figure 5. Percentage of adults aged 19–25 with health insurance, by coverage type, and percentage uninsured at the time of interview: United States, 1997–2012

NOTE: Data are based on household interviews of a sample of the civilian noninstitutionalized population.

DATA SOURCE: CDC/NCHS, National Health Interview Survey, 1997–2012, Family Core component.

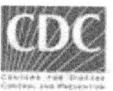

addition, for ages 18–64, 20.2% of poor adults, 37.2% of near-poor adults, and 81.3% of not-poor adults were covered by private health insurance.

Lack of coverage, by selected demographic characteristics

Race/ethnicity

Based on data from the 2012 NHIS, Hispanic persons were more likely than non-Hispanic white, non-Hispanic black, and non-Hispanic Asian persons to be uninsured at the time of interview, to have been uninsured for at least part of the past 12 months, and to have been uninsured for more than a year (Table 7). More than one-quarter of Hispanic persons were uninsured at the time of interview, and one-third had been uninsured for at least part of the past year.

Age and sex

Based on data from the 2012 NHIS, adults aged 25–34 were the most likely to lack health insurance coverage at the time of interview (28.2%) (Table 7). Among adults in age groups 18–24, 25–34, 35–44, and 45-64, men were more likely than women to lack health insurance coverage at the time of interview (Figure 2).

Other demographic characteristics

Based on data from the 2012 NHIS, lack of health insurance coverage was greatest in the South and West regions of the United States (Table 7).

Among adults who lacked a high school diploma, 32.1% were uninsured at the time of interview, 36.0% had been uninsured for at least part of the past year, and 27.5% had been uninsured for more than a year at the time of interview. These rates are two to more than three times as high as those for persons with more than a high school education.

Among currently unemployed adults aged 18–64, 54.2% had been uninsured for at least part of the past year and 33.3% had been uninsured for

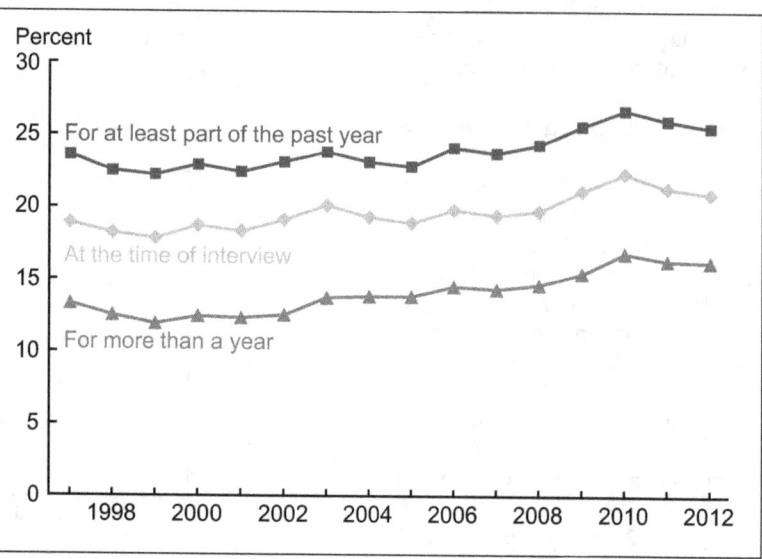

Figure 6. Percentages of adults aged 18–64 who lacked health insurance coverage at the time of interview, for at least part of the past year, or for more than a year: United States, 1997–2012

NOTE: Data are based on household interviews of a sample of the civilian noninstitutionalized population.

DATA SOURCE: CDC/NCHS, National Health Interview Survey, 1997–2012, Family Core component.

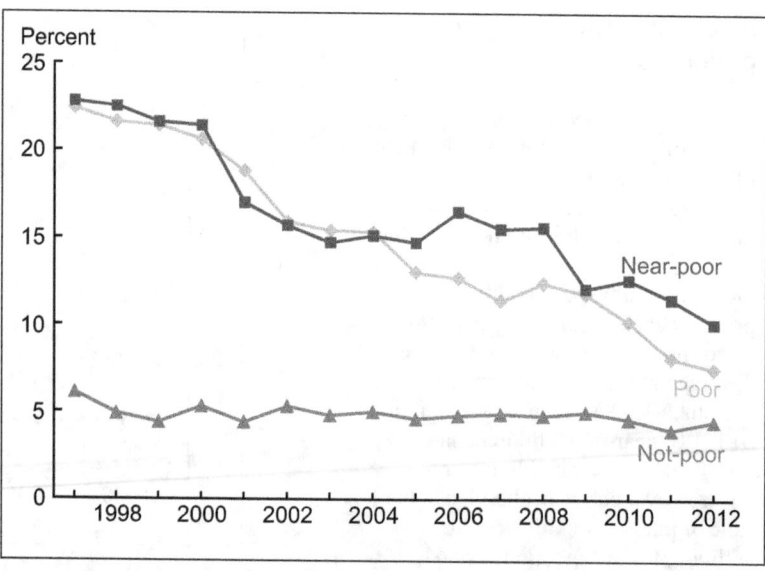

Figure 7. Percentage of children under age 18 who were uninsured at the time of interview, by poverty status: United States, 1997–2012

NOTE: Data are based on household interviews of a sample of the civilian noninstitutionalized population.

DATA SOURCE: CDC/NCHS, National Health Interview Survey, 1997–2012, Family Core component.

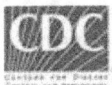

more than a year. Among employed adults in the same age group, 22.9% had been uninsured for at least part of the past year and 14.8% had been uninsured for more than a year. Married or widowed adults aged 18 and over were more likely to have coverage than those who were divorced, separated, living with a partner, or never married.

Quarterly and annual estimates for adults aged 19–25 and 26–35

Among adults aged 19–25, the percentage uninsured decreased from 35.6% in the third quarter of 2010 (a recent high point in uninsurance) to 27.0% in the fourth quarter of 2012 (Table 8). There was a corresponding increase in private coverage for this age group, from 49.3% in the third quarter of 2010 (a recent low point in private coverage) to 57.9% in the fourth quarter of 2012.

Among adults aged 26–35, the percentage who were uninsured was the same in the third quarter of 2010 and the fourth quarter of 2012 (27.7%). The change in private coverage for this age group (from 59.5% in the third quarter of 2010 to 58.8% in the fourth quarter of 2012) was not significantly different.

Quarterly and annual estimates for adults aged 19–25, by selected demographic characteristics

Among both male and female adults aged 19–25, there was a decrease in the percentage uninsured between the third quarter of 2010 and the fourth quarter of 2012 (Table 9).

For 2012, the percentage uninsured ranged from 18.2% in the Northeast to 31.2% in the South (Table 10). Hispanic adults had the highest percentage uninsured (46.6%), compared with non-Hispanic black (30.1%) and non-Hispanic white (18.4%) adults (Table 11).

Estimates of enrollment in HDHPs, CDHPs, and FSAs

Based on data from the 2012 NHIS, 31.1% of persons under age 65 with private health insurance were

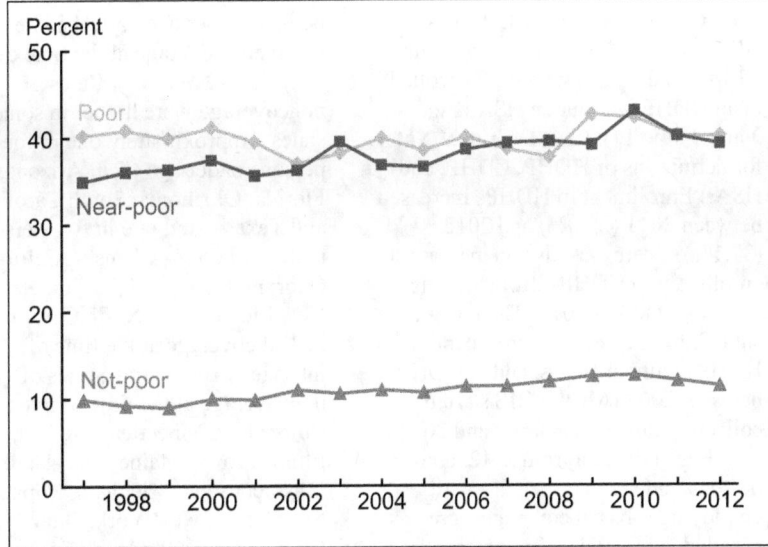

Figure 8. Percentage of adults aged 18–64 who were uninsured at the time of interview, by poverty status: United States, 1997–2012

NOTE: Data are based on household interviews of a sample of the civilian noninstitutionalized population.

DATA SOURCE: CDC/NCHS, National Health Interview Survey, 1997–2012, Family Core component.

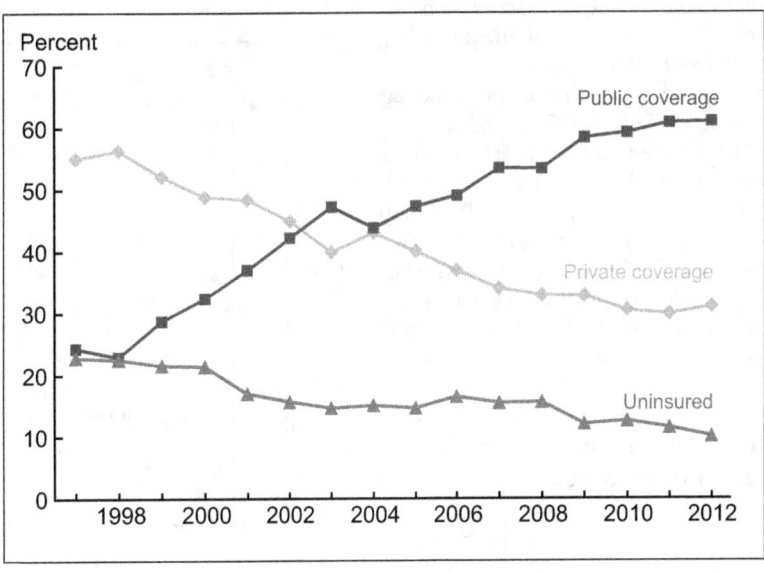

Figure 9. Percentage of near-poor children under age 18 with health insurance, by coverage type, and percentage uninsured at the time of interview: United States, 1997–2012

NOTE: Data are based on household interviews of a sample of the civilian noninstitutionalized population.

DATA SOURCE: CDC/NCHS, National Health Interview Survey, 1997–2012, Family Core component.

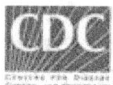

enrolled in an HDHP, including 10.8% who were enrolled in a CDHP [an HDHP with a health savings account (HSA)] and 20.3% who were enrolled in an HDHP without an HSA (**Figure 3** and **Table 12**). (See **Technical Notes** for definitions of HDHP, CDHP, and HSA.) Enrollment in HDHPs increased between 2011 (29.0%) and 2012 (31.1%). There was also an increase in enrollment in CDHPs, from 9.2% in 2011 to 10.8% in 2012. There was a significant increase in enrollment in HDHPs without HSAs, and in CDHPs, between 2007 (when NHIS started collecting this information) and 2012.

Based on data from 2012, among persons under age 65, 29.2% with employment-based coverage were enrolled in an HDHP, an increase from 26.9% in 2011 and 15.6% in 2007 (**Table 13**). Among persons under age 65, 54.7% with directly purchased private health plans were enrolled in an HDHP, an increase from 39.2% in 2007. For persons under age 65, approximately 8% of private health plans were directly purchased (estimates not shown). HDHPs constitute a growing share of both employment-based and directly purchased health plans.

In 2012, among persons under age 65 with private health insurance, 21.6% were in a family that had an FSA for medical expenses (**Table 12**). (See **Technical Notes** for definition of FSA.) This is an increase from 2007, when 16.7% were in a family with an FSA. However, there has been no significant increase in FSA enrollment since 2009.

Insurance coverage in selected states

State-specific health insurance estimates are presented for 43 states for persons of all ages, persons under age 65, and adults aged 18–64. State-specific estimates are presented for 38 states for children aged 0–17. Estimates are not presented for all 50 states and the District of Columbia due to considerations of sample size and precision.

Nationally in 2012, 16.9% of persons under age 65 lacked health insurance coverage at the time of interview (**Table 14**). Rates of noncoverage were higher in some states. Approximately one in four persons under age 65 in Arizona, Florida, Oklahoma, South Carolina, and Texas—and one in five persons under age 65 in Arkansas, California, Georgia, Idaho, Mississippi, Nevada, New Mexico, and North Carolina—lacked coverage at the time of interview. By contrast, rates of noncoverage at the time of interview in Colorado, Connecticut, Hawaii, Illinois, Iowa, Maine, Maryland, Massachusetts, Michigan, Minnesota, New Jersey, New York, Ohio, Pennsylvania, Rhode Island, and Virginia were significantly lower than the national average (16.9%).

In the U.S. overall, 6.6% of children in 2012 lacked coverage at the time of interview, but rates were significantly higher in Arizona (15.6%), Florida (9.6%), Nevada (12.2%), South Carolina (13.8%), Texas (11.0%), and Utah (10.7%).

Nationally, 42.1% of children had public health care coverage. Among the 38 states examined for this report, public coverage for children ranged from 22.7% in Minnesota to 59.1% in Mississippi.

In the U.S. overall, 61.0% of persons under age 65 had private coverage. Among the 43 states examined, private coverage rates for this age group ranged from 41.6% in New Mexico to 78.0% in Minnesota. Colorado, Connecticut, Illinois, Iowa, Kansas, Maryland, Massachusetts, Michigan, Minnesota, Nebraska, New Jersey, Ohio, Pennsylvania, Utah, Virginia, and Wisconsin had rates significantly above the national average.

Long-term trends in coverage

Lack of health insurance coverage

The percentage of children uninsured at the time of interview decreased from 13.9% in 1997 to 8.9% in 2005. Between 2005 and 2008, the

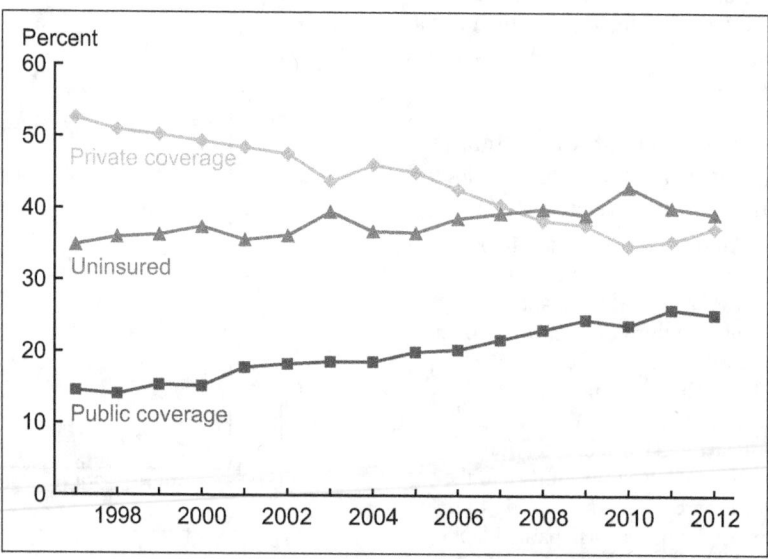

Figure 10. Percentage of near-poor adults aged 18–64 with health insurance, by coverage type, and percentage uninsured at the time of interview: United States, 1997–2012

NOTE: Data are based on household interviews of a sample of the civilian noninstitutionalized population.

DATA SOURCE: CDC/NCHS, National Health Interview Survey, 1997–2012, Family Core component.

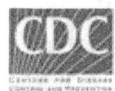

percentage remained relatively stable, ranging from 8.9% in 2005, 2007, and 2008, to 9.3% in 2006. Since 2008, the percentage has decreased from 8.9% to 6.6% in 2012 (Figure 4).

Since 1997, the percentage of adults aged 18–64 who were uninsured at the time of interview was lowest in 1999 (17.8%) and highest in 2010 (22.3%) (Table 1). More recently, there was a decrease in the percentage, from 22.3% in 2010 to 20.9% in 2012. Prior to this recent decrease, the percentage had generally been increasing since 1997.

Since 1997, the percentage of adults aged 19–25 who were uninsured at the time of interview was lowest in 2012 (26.4%) and highest in 2010 (33.9%) (Figure 5). Prior to this recent decrease, the percentage had generally been increasing since 1997.

The percentage of children who were uninsured during at least part of the year prior to interview decreased from 18.1% in 1997 to 12.6% in 2005. Between 2005 and 2008, the percentage remained relatively stable and ranged between 12.6% in 2005 and 2007 and 13.3% in 2008. Since 2008, the percentage has decreased from 13.3% in 2008 to 10.4% in 2012 (Figure 4).

From 1997 through 2012, the percentage of adults aged 18–64 who lacked coverage for at least part of the year prior to interview was lowest in 1999 (22.2%) and highest in 2010 (26.7%) (Figure 6). More recently, the percentage decreased from 26.7% in 2010 to 25.5% in 2012.

Among adults aged 18–64, between 1997 and 2012, the percentage uninsured for more than a year was lowest in 1999 (11.9%) and highest in 2010 (16.8%) (Figure 6).

The percentage of children uninsured for more than a year decreased from 8.4% in 1997 to 3.7% in 2012 (Figure 4).

Public and private coverage

Public coverage rates among children and among adults aged 18–64 were higher in 2012 than in 1997. However, the increase among adults was smaller than the increase among children (Table 3). Public coverage for

children more than doubled, from 20.0% in 1998 to 42.1% in 2012. Conversely, private health care coverage rates among children and among adults aged 18–64 were lower in 2012 than in 1997. Among adults aged 19–25, public coverage increased from 9.1% in 2000 to 17.5% in 2012. Private coverage has generally decreased since 1999 but, as noted previously, the percentage with private coverage increased between 2010 and 2012 for those aged 19–25 (Figure 5).

Insurance coverage, by poverty status

The percentage of poor children who were uninsured at the time of interview decreased from 1997 through 2012 (Figure 7). During the same period, the percentage of poor adults who were uninsured remained relatively stable (Figure 8).

Among children, all poverty status groups experienced an increase in public coverage between 1997 and the 2012 (Table 5). However, the largest increase was seen among near-poor children, for whom coverage by a public plan increased by 36.7 percentage points during the same period.

The rate of private coverage among near-poor children was 23.9 percentage points lower in 2012 than in 1997 (Table 6). As shown in Figure 9, among near-poor children, the percentage without health insurance and the percentage with private health insurance coverage have declined since 1997, while public coverage increased.

Private coverage generally decreased among near-poor adults aged 18–64—from 52.6% in 1997 to 37.2% in 2012—so that the uninsured rate in 2012 was higher than the private coverage rate for this population during the same period (Figure 10). Among not-poor adults aged 18–64, private coverage generally decreased from 1997 through 2012 (Table 6).

References

1. U.S. Government Accountability Office. Consumer-directed health plans: Early enrollee experiences with health savings accounts and eligible health plans. GAO–06–798. Washington, DC: GAO. 2006.

2. Joinpoint Regression Program, version 3.4 [computer software]. Bethesda, MD: Statistical Research and Applications Branch, National Cancer Institute. 2009.

3. Cohen RA, Martinez ME. Impact of Medicare and Medicaid probe questions on health insurance estimates from the National Health Interview Survey, 2004. Health E-Stat. National Center for Health Statistics. 2005. Available from: http://www.cdc.gov/nchs/data/hestat/impact04/impact04.htm.

4. Lamison-White L. Poverty in the United States, 1996. U.S. Bureau of the Census. Current population reports, P60–198. Washington, DC: U.S. Government Printing Office. 1997.

5. Dalaker J, Naifeh M. Poverty in the United States, 1997. U.S. Bureau of the Census. Current population reports, P60–201. Washington, DC: U.S. Government Printing Office. 1998.

6. Dalaker J. Poverty in the United States, 1998. U.S. Census Bureau. Current population reports, P60–207. Washington, DC: U.S. Government Printing Office. 1999.

7. Dalaker J, Proctor BD. Poverty in the United States, 1999. U.S. Census Bureau. Current population reports, P60–210. Washington, DC: U.S. Government Printing Office. 2000.

8. Dalaker J. Poverty in the United States, 2000. U.S. Census Bureau. Current population reports, P60–214. Washington, DC: U.S. Government Printing Office. 2001.

9. Proctor BD, Dalaker J. Poverty in the United States, 2001. U.S. Census Bureau. Current population reports, P60–219.

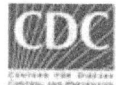

Washington, DC: U.S. Government Printing Office. 2002.

10. Proctor BD, Dalaker J. Poverty in the United States, 2002. U.S. Census Bureau. Current population reports, P60–222. Washington, DC: U.S. Government Printing Office. 2003.

11. DeNavas-Walt C, Proctor BD, Mills RJ. Income, poverty, and health insurance coverage in the United States: 2003. U.S. Census Bureau. Current population reports, P60–226. Washington, DC: U.S. Government Printing Office. 2004.

12. DeNavas-Walt C, Proctor BD, Lee CH. Income, poverty, and health insurance coverage in the United States: 2004. U.S. Census Bureau. Current population reports, P60–229. Washington, DC: U.S. Government Printing Office. 2005.

13. DeNavas-Walt C, Proctor BD, Lee CH. Income, poverty, and health insurance coverage in the United States: 2005. U.S. Census Bureau. Current population reports, P60–231. Washington, DC: U.S. Government Printing Office. 2006.

14. DeNavas-Walt C, Proctor BD, Smith J. Income, poverty, and health insurance coverage in the United States: 2006. U.S. Census Bureau. Current population reports, P60–233. Washington, DC: U.S. Government Printing Office. 2007.

15. DeNavas-Walt C, Proctor BD, Smith JC. Income, poverty, and health insurance coverage in the United States: 2007. U.S. Census Bureau. Current population reports, P60–235. Washington, DC: U.S. Government Printing Office. 2008.

16. DeNavas-Walt C, Proctor BD, Smith JC. Income, poverty, and health insurance coverage in the United States: 2008. U.S. Census Bureau. Current population reports, P60–236. Washington, DC: U.S. Government Printing Office. 2009.

17. DeNavas-Walt C, Proctor BD, Smith JC. Income, poverty, and health insurance coverage in the United States: 2009. U.S. Census Bureau. Current population reports, P60–238. Washington, DC: U.S. Government Printing Office. 2010.

18. DeNavas-Walt C, Proctor BD, Smith JC. Income, poverty, and health insurance coverage in the United States: 2010. U.S. Census Bureau. Current population reports, P60–239. Washington, DC: U.S. Government Printing Office. 2011.

19. DeNavas-Walt C, Proctor BD, Smith JC. Income, poverty, and health insurance coverage in the United States: 2011. U.S. Census Bureau. Current population reports, P60–243. Washington, DC: U.S. Government Printing Office. 2012.

20. Pleis JR, Dahlhamer JM, Meyer PS. Unfolding the answers? Income nonresponse and income brackets in the National Health Interview Survey. Proceedings of the 2006 Joint Statistical Meetings [CD–ROM]. Alexandria, VA: American Statistical Association; 3540–47. 2007.

21. Pleis JR, Cohen RA. Impact of income bracketing on poverty measures used in the National Health Interview Survey's Early Release Program: Preliminary data from the 2007 NHIS. Hyattsville, MD: National Center for Health Statistics. 2007. Available from: http://www.cdc.gov/nchs/data/nhis/income.pdf.

22. National Center for Health Statistics. Health, United States, 2011: With special feature on socioeconomic status and health. Hyattsville, MD. 2012. Available from: http://www.cdc.gov/nchs/hus.htm.

23. Schiller JS, Ward BW, Freeman G, Peregoy JA. Early release of selected estimates based on data from the 2012 National Health Interview Survey. National Center for Health Statistics. June 2013. Available from: http://www.cdc.gov/nchs/nhis.htm.

24. Blumberg SJ, Luke JV. Wireless substitution: Early release of estimates based on data from the National Health Interview Survey, July–December 2012. National Center for Health Statistics. June 2013. Available from: http://www.cdc.gov/nchs/nhis.htm.

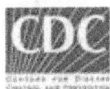

Table 1. Percentages of persons who lacked health insurance coverage at the time of interview, for at least part of the past year, and for more than a year, by age group: United States, 1997–2012

Age group and year	Uninsured[1] at the time of interview	Uninsured[1] for at least part of the past year[2]	Uninsured[1] for more than a year[2]
	Percent (standard error)		
All ages			
1997	15.4 (0.21)	19.5 (0.24)	10.4 (0.18)
1998	14.6 (0.23)	18.6 (0.26)	9.8 (0.19)
1999	14.2 (0.22)	18.2 (0.25)	9.3 (0.19)
2000	14.9 (0.22)	18.7 (0.24)	9.6 (0.18)
2001	14.3 (0.23)	18.0 (0.26)	9.3 (0.18)
2002	14.7 (0.22)	18.3 (0.24)	9.3 (0.17)
2003	15.2 (0.24)	18.6 (0.26)	10.0 (0.19)
2004 (Method 1)[3]	14.7 (0.21)	18.0 (0.23)	10.1 (0.17)
2004 (Method 2)[3]	14.6 (0.20)	17.9 (0.23)	10.1 (0.17)
2005[3]	14.2 (0.21)	17.6 (0.23)	10.0 (0.18)
2006[3,4]	14.8 (0.26)	18.6 (0.29)	10.5 (0.22)
2007[3]	14.5 (0.29)	18.2 (0.34)	10.3 (0.24)
2008[3]	14.7 (0.32)	18.7 (0.33)	10.6 (0.26)
2009[3]	15.4 (0.30)	19.4 (0.32)	10.9 (0.26)
2010[3]	16.0 (0.27)	19.8 (0.29)	11.7 (0.22)
2011[3]	15.1 (0.25)	19.2 (0.29)	11.2 (0.21)
2012[3]	14.7 (0.23)	18.6 (0.27)	11.1 (0.22)
Under 65 years			
1997	17.4 (0.24)	21.9 (0.28)	11.8 (0.21)
1998	16.5 (0.26)	20.9 (0.29)	11.0 (0.21)
1999	16.0 (0.25)	20.4 (0.28)	10.5 (0.21)
2000	16.8 (0.24)	21.0 (0.26)	10.8 (0.20)
2001	16.2 (0.26)	20.3 (0.29)	10.5 (0.21)
2002	16.5 (0.24)	20.6 (0.27)	10.4 (0.19)
2003	17.2 (0.27)	20.9 (0.28)	11.2 (0.21)
2004 (Method 1)[3]	16.6 (0.23)	20.2 (0.26)	11.4 (0.19)
2004 (Method 2)[3]	16.4 (0.23)	20.1 (0.26)	11.4 (0.19)
2005[3]	16.0 (0.24)	19.9 (0.26)	11.3 (0.21)
2006[3,4]	16.8 (0.29)	20.9 (0.32)	11.8 (0.25)
2007[3]	16.4 (0.33)	20.5 (0.38)	11.7 (0.27)
2008[3]	16.7 (0.36)	21.2 (0.37)	12.0 (0.29)
2009[3]	17.5 (0.34)	22.0 (0.36)	12.4 (0.29)
2010[3]	18.2 (0.30)	22.5 (0.33)	13.3 (0.24)
2011[3]	17.3 (0.29)	21.8 (0.33)	12.7 (0.25)
2012[3]	16.9 (0.27)	21.3 (0.31)	12.7 (0.24)

See footnotes at end of table.

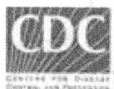

Table 1. Percentages of persons who lacked health insurance coverage at the time of interview, for at least part of the past year, and for more than a year, by age group: United States, 1997–2012 (cont.)

Age group and year	Uninsured[1] at the time of interview	Uninsured[1] for at least part of the past year[2]	Uninsured[1] for more than a year[2]
	Percent (standard error)		
0–17 years			
1997	13.9 (0.36)	18.1 (0.41)	8.4 (0.29)
1998	12.7 (0.34)	17.1 (0.40)	7.6 (0.27)
1999	11.8 (0.32)	16.3 (0.39)	7.2 (0.26)
2000	12.3 (0.32)	16.7 (0.35)	7.0 (0.23)
2001	11.0 (0.34)	15.2 (0.41)	6.3 (0.25)
2002	10.5 (0.32)	14.6 (0.37)	5.6 (0.24)
2003	10.1 (0.34)	13.7 (0.37)	5.3 (0.25)
2004 (Method 1)[3]	9.6 (0.29)	12.9 (0.33)	5.4 (0.25)
2004 (Method 2)[3]	9.4 (0.29)	12.7 (0.33)	5.4 (0.25)
2005[3]	8.9 (0.29)	12.6 (0.33)	5.3 (0.24)
2006[3,4]	9.3 (0.34)	13.0 (0.40)	5.2 (0.26)
2007[3]	8.9 (0.40)	12.6 (0.48)	5.0 (0.28)
2008[3]	8.9 (0.43)	13.3 (0.49)	5.6 (0.35)
2009[3]	8.2 (0.40)	12.8 (0.47)	4.8 (0.31)
2010[3]	7.8 (0.32)	11.6 (0.37)	4.5 (0.23)
2011[3]	7.0 (0.27)	10.9 (0.36)	3.7 (0.19)
2012[3]	6.6 (0.27)	10.4 (0.35)	3.7 (0.19)
18–64 years			
1997	18.9 (0.23)	23.6 (0.26)	13.3 (0.21)
1998	18.2 (0.27)	22.5 (0.30)	12.5 (0.23)
1999	17.8 (0.26)	22.2 (0.29)	11.9 (0.23)
2000	18.7 (0.27)	22.9 (0.29)	12.4 (0.23)
2001	18.3 (0.27)	22.4 (0.29)	12.3 (0.22)
2002	19.1 (0.26)	23.1 (0.29)	12.5 (0.21)
2003	20.1 (0.29)	23.8 (0.31)	13.7 (0.25)
2004 (Method 1)[3]	19.4 (0.26)	23.2 (0.29)	13.8 (0.21)
2004 (Method 2)[3]	19.3 (0.26)	23.1 (0.29)	13.8 (0.21)
2005[3]	18.9 (0.26)	22.8 (0.28)	13.8 (0.23)
2006[3,4]	19.8 (0.33)	24.1 (0.36)	14.5 (0.29)
2007[3]	19.4 (0.36)	23.7 (0.40)	14.3 (0.32)
2008[3]	19.7 (0.40)	24.3 (0.40)	14.6 (0.34)
2009[3]	21.1 (0.37)	25.6 (0.38)	15.4 (0.34)
2010[3]	22.3 (0.35)	26.7 (0.37)	16.8 (0.30)
2011[3]	21.3 (0.34)	26.0 (0.37)	16.3 (0.31)
2012[3]	20.9 (0.31)	25.5 (0.34)	16.2 (0.29)

See footnotes at end of table.

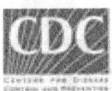

Table 1. Percentages of persons who lacked health insurance coverage at the time of interview, for at least part of the past year, and for more than a year, by age group: United States, 1997–2012 (cont.)

Age group and year	Uninsured[1] at the time of interview	Uninsured[1] for at least part of the past year[2]	Uninsured[1] for more than a year[2]
	Percent (standard error)		
19–25 years			
1997	31.4 (0.63)	39.2 (0.67)	20.8 (0.51)
1998	29.8 (0.68)	37.8 (0.76)	20.2 (0.62)
1999	29.4 (0.66)	36.9 (0.73)	18.2 (0.53)
2000	31.4 (0.74)	39.4 (0.78)	19.7 (0.57)
2001	30.8 (0.66)	37.4 (0.69)	20.0 (0.56)
2002	29.4 (0.74)	36.7 (0.83)	19.0 (0.58)
2003	32.0 (0.74)	38.4 (0.77)	21.5 (0.63)
2004 (Method 1)[3]	32.2 (0.69)	38.9 (0.71)	21.7 (0.60)
2004 (Method 2)[3]	32.1 (0.69)	38.8 (0.71)	21.7 (0.60)
2005[3]	31.2 (0.65)	37.9 (0.68)	21.6 (0.54)
2006[3,4]	32.3 (0.84)	39.8 (0.91)	22.3 (0.72)
2007[3]	30.2 (0.86)	37.5 (0.93)	20.5 (0.73)
2008[3]	30.9 (0.87)	39.1 (0.91)	21.2 (0.74)
2009[3]	32.7 (0.82)	40.3 (0.87)	22.0 (0.74)
2010[3]	33.9 (0.73)	41.7 (0.78)	24.1 (0.61)
2011[3]	27.9 (0.71)	36.1 (0.77)	20.1 (0.61)
2012[3]	26.4 (0.72)	33.0 (0.72)	19.6 (0.62)

[1]A person was defined as uninsured if he or she did not have any private health insurance, Medicare, Medicaid, Children's Health Insurance Program (CHIP), state-sponsored or other government-sponsored health plan, or military plan. A person was also defined as uninsured if he or she had only Indian Health Service coverage or had only a private plan that paid for one type of service, such as accidents or dental care.

[2]A year is defined as the 12 months prior to interview.

[3]Beginning in the third quarter of 2004, two additional questions were added to the National Health Interview Survey (NHIS) insurance section to reduce potential errors in reporting Medicare and Medicaid status. Persons aged 65 and over not reporting Medicare coverage were asked explicitly about Medicare coverage, and persons under age 65 with no reported coverage were asked explicitly about Medicaid coverage. Estimates of uninsurance for 2004 were calculated both without the additional information from these questions (noted as Method 1) and with the responses to these questions (noted as Method 2). Respondents who were reclassified as "covered" by the additional questions received the appropriate follow-up questions concerning periods of noncoverage for insured respondents. These reclassified respondents were excluded in the tabulation of "Uninsured for more than a year" using Method 1 in 2004. Beginning in 2005, all estimates were calculated using Method 2. See Technical Notes for additional information.

[4]In 2006, NHIS underwent a sample redesign. The impact of the new sample design on estimates presented in this report is minimal.

NOTE: Data are based on household interviews of a sample of the civilian noninstitutionalized population.

DATA SOURCE: CDC/NCHS, National Health Interview Survey, 1997–2012, Family Core component.

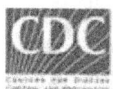

Table 2. Numbers of persons who lacked health insurance coverage at the time of interview, for at least part of the past year, and for more than a year, by age group: United States, 1997–2012

Age group and year	Uninsured[1] at the time of interview	Uninsured[1] for at least part of the past year[2]	Uninsured[1] for more than a year[2]
	Number in millions		
All ages			
1997	41.0	51.9	27.7
1998	39.3	49.9	26.3
1999	38.7	49.4	25.3
2000	41.3	51.8	26.6
2001	40.2	50.4	26.1
2002	41.5	51.7	26.2
2003	43.6	53.1	28.5
2004 (Method 1)[3]	42.5	52.0	29.2
2004 (Method 2)[3]	42.1	51.6	29.2
2005[3]	41.2	51.3	29.2
2006[3,4]	43.6	54.5	30.7
2007[3]	43.1	53.9	30.6
2008[3]	43.8	55.9	31.7
2009[3]	46.3	58.5	32.8
2010[3]	48.6	60.3	35.7
2011[3]	46.3	58.7	34.2
2012[3]	45.5	57.7	34.1
Under 65 years			
1997	40.7	51.4	27.6
1998	39.0	49.5	26.2
1999	38.3	48.9	25.1
2000	40.8	51.3	26.4
2001	39.8	49.9	25.9
2002	41.1	51.2	25.9
2003	43.2	52.5	28.3
2004 (Method 1)[3]	42.0	51.3	28.9
2004 (Method 2)[3]	41.7	51.0	28.9
2005[3]	41.0	50.9	29.0
2006[3,4]	43.3	54.0	30.5
2007[3]	42.8	53.5	30.4
2008[3]	43.6	55.5	31.6
2009[3]	46.0	57.9	32.6
2010[3]	48.2	59.6	35.4
2011[3]	45.9	58.0	33.9
2012[3]	45.2	56.8	33.9

See footnotes at end of table.

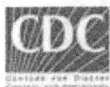

Table 2. Numbers of persons who lacked health insurance coverage at the time of interview, for at least part of the past year, and for more than a year, by age group: United States, 1997–2012 (cont.)

Age group and year	Uninsured[1] at the time of interview	Uninsured[1] for at least part of the past year[2]	Uninsured[1] for more than a year[2]
	Number in millions		
0–17 years			
1997	9.9	12.9	6.0
1998	9.1	12.3	5.5
1999	8.5	11.8	5.2
2000	8.9	12.0	5.1
2001	7.9	11.0	4.5
2002	7.6	10.6	4.1
2003	7.3	10.0	3.9
2004 (Method 1)[3]	7.0	9.4	4.0
2004 (Method 2)[3]	6.8	9.3	3.9
2005[3]	6.5	9.3	3.9
2006[3,4]	6.8	9.5	3.8
2007[3]	6.5	9.3	3.7
2008[3]	6.6	9.9	4.1
2009[3]	6.1	9.5	3.6
2010[3]	5.8	8.7	3.4
2011[3]	5.2	8.1	2.7
2012[3]	4.9	7.7	2.7
18–64 years			
1997	30.8	38.5	21.7
1998	30.0	37.2	20.7
1999	29.8	37.1	19.9
2000	32.0	39.2	21.3
2001	31.9	38.9	21.4
2002	33.5	40.6	21.9
2003	35.9	42.5	24.5
2004 (Method 1)[3]	35.0	41.9	25.0
2004 (Method 2)[3]	34.9	41.8	25.0
2005[3]	34.5	41.7	25.2
2006[3,4]	36.5	44.5	26.8
2007[3]	36.3	44.2	26.8
2008[3]	37.1	45.6	27.5
2009[3]	40.0	48.4	29.1
2010[3]	42.5	51.0	32.0
2011[3]	40.7	49.9	31.2
2012[3]	40.3	49.2	31.2

See footnotes at end of table.

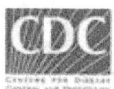

Table 2. Numbers of persons who lacked health insurance coverage at the time of interview, for at least part of the past year, and for more than a year, by age group: United States, 1997–2012 (cont.)

Age group and year	Uninsured[1] at the time of interview	Uninsured[1] for at least part of the past year[2]	Uninsured[1] for more than a year[2]
	Number in millions		
19–25 years			
1997	7.7	9.7	5.1
1998	7.4	9.3	5.0
1999	7.3	9.2	4.5
2000	8.1	10.2	5.1
2001	8.1	9.9	5.3
2002	7.9	9.8	5.1
2003	8.9	10.6	6.0
2004 (Method 1)[3]	8.9	10.8	6.1
2004 (Method 2)[3]	8.9	10.8	6.1
2005[3]	8.8	10.7	6.1
2006[3,4]	9.3	11.4	6.4
2007[3]	8.8	10.9	6.0
2008[3]	8.9	11.2	6.1
2009[3]	9.5	11.6	6.4
2010[3]	10.0	12.3	7.1
2011[3]	8.4	10.8	6.0
2012[3]	7.9	9.9	5.9

[1]A person was defined as uninsured if he or she did not have any private health insurance, Medicare, Medicaid, Children's Health Insurance Program (CHIP), state-sponsored or other government-sponsored health plan, or military plan. A person was also defined as uninsured if he or she had only Indian Health Service coverage or had only a private plan that paid for one type of service, such as accidents or dental care.

[2]A year is defined as the 12 months prior to interview.

[3]Beginning in the third quarter of 2004, two additional questions were added to the National Health Interview Survey (NHIS) insurance section to reduce potential errors in reporting Medicare and Medicaid status. Persons aged 65 and over not reporting Medicare coverage were asked explicitly about Medicare coverage, and persons under age 65 with no reported coverage were asked explicitly about Medicaid coverage. Estimates of uninsurance for 2004 were calculated both without the additional information from these questions (noted as Method 1) and with the responses to these questions (noted as Method 2). Respondents who were reclassified as "covered" by the additional questions received the appropriate follow-up questions concerning periods of noncoverage for insured respondents. These reclassified respondents were excluded in the tabulation of "Uninsured for more than a year" using Method 1 in 2004. Beginning in 2005, all estimates were calculated using Method 2. See Technical Notes for additional information.

[4]In 2006, NHIS underwent a sample redesign. The impact of the new sample design on estimates presented in this report is minimal.

NOTE: Data are based on household interviews of a sample of the civilian noninstitutionalized population.

DATA SOURCE: CDC/NCHS, National Health Interview Survey, 1997–2012, Family Core component.

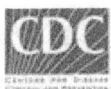

Table 3. Percentages of persons under age 65 with public health plan coverage and with private health insurance coverage, at the time of interview, by age group: United States, 1997–2012

Type of coverage and year	Age group			
	Under 65 years	0–17 years	18–64 years	19–25 years
	Percent (standard error)			
Public health plan coverage[1]				
1997	13.6 (0.25)	21.4 (0.48)	10.2 (0.20)	11.2 (0.46)
1998	12.7 (0.26)	20.0 (0.49)	9.5 (0.21)	9.8 (0.42)
1999	12.4 (0.24)	20.4 (0.46)	9.0 (0.19)	9.5 (0.40)
2000	12.9 (0.26)	22.0 (0.50)	9.1 (0.19)	9.1 (0.42)
2001	13.6 (0.26)	23.6 (0.50)	9.4 (0.21)	9.6 (0.42)
2002	15.2 (0.29)	27.1 (0.54)	10.3 (0.23)	10.9 (0.45)
2003	16.0 (0.31)	28.6 (0.58)	10.9 (0.24)	11.1 (0.42)
2004 (Method 1)[2]	16.1 (0.29)	28.5 (0.54)	11.1 (0.22)	11.5 (0.42)
2004 (Method 2)[2]	16.2 (0.29)	28.7 (0.54)	11.1 (0.23)	11.6 (0.42)
2005[2]	16.8 (0.29)	29.9 (0.56)	11.5 (0.22)	12.9 (0.51)
2006[2,3]	18.1 (0.35)	32.3 (0.69)	12.4 (0.26)	12.3 (0.50)
2007[2]	18.1 (0.40)	32.7 (0.77)	12.3 (0.31)	12.3 (0.56)
2008[2]	19.3 (0.42)	34.2 (0.79)	13.4 (0.33)	14.0 (0.75)
2009[2]	21.0 (0.39)	37.7 (0.76)	14.4 (0.31)	15.0 (0.62)
2010[2]	22.0 (0.38)	39.8 (0.73)	15.0 (0.30)	15.7 (0.55)
2011[3]	23.0 (0.37)	41.0 (0.74)	15.9 (0.29)	16.8 (0.60)
2012[3]	23.5 (0.37)	42.1 (0.72)	16.4 (0.29)	17.5 (0.59)
Private health insurance coverage[4]				
1997	70.8 (0.35)	66.2 (0.57)	72.8 (0.30)	58.4 (0.71)
1998	72.0 (0.36)	68.5 (0.55)	73.5 (0.32)	59.5 (0.71)
1999	73.1 (0.36)	69.1 (0.55)	74.7 (0.33)	61.8 (0.73)
2000	71.8 (0.34)	67.1 (0.53)	73.8 (0.32)	60.2 (0.75)
2001	71.6 (0.37)	66.7 (0.57)	73.7 (0.33)	60.4 (0.73)
2002	69.8 (0.39)	63.9 (0.61)	72.3 (0.35)	60.6 (0.86)
2003	68.2 (0.40)	62.6 (0.60)	70.6 (0.36)	57.7 (0.86)
2004[2]	68.6 (0.39)	63.1 (0.59)	70.9 (0.36)	57.1 (0.77)
2005[2]	68.4 (0.39)	62.4 (0.60)	70.9 (0.36)	56.5 (0.79)
2006[2,3]	66.5 (0.48)	59.7 (0.72)	69.2 (0.43)	56.0 (0.96)
2007[2]	66.8 (0.53)	59.9 (0.82)	69.6 (0.47)	58.1 (1.00)
2008[2]	65.4 (0.57)	58.3 (0.84)	68.1 (0.54)	55.7 (1.02)
2009[2]	62.9 (0.54)	55.7 (0.86)	65.8 (0.47)	52.6 (0.91)
2010[2]	61.2 (0.50)	53.8 (0.75)	64.1 (0.46)	51.0 (0.84)
2011[3]	61.2 (0.51)	53.3 (0.76)	64.2 (0.45)	56.2 (0.85)
2012[3]	61.0 (0.47)	52.8 (0.73)	64.1 (0.42)	57.2 (0.85)

[1]Includes Medicaid, Children's Health Insurance Program (CHIP), state-sponsored or other government-sponsored health plan, Medicare (disability), and military plans.
[2]Beginning in the third quarter of 2004, two additional questions were added to the National Health Interview Survey (NHIS) insurance section to reduce potential errors in reporting Medicare and Medicaid status. Persons aged 65 and over not reporting Medicare coverage were asked explicitly about Medicare coverage, and persons under age 65 with no reported coverage were asked explicitly about Medicaid coverage. Estimates of uninsurance for 2004 were calculated both without the additional information from these questions (noted as Method 1) and with the responses to these questions (noted as Method 2). Respondents who were reclassified as "covered" by the additional questions received the appropriate follow-up questions concerning periods of noncoverage for insured respondents. The two additional questions added beginning in the third quarter of 2004 did not affect the estimates of private coverage. Beginning in 2005, all estimates were calculated using Method 2. See Technical Notes for additional information.
[3]In 2006, NHIS underwent a sample redesign. The impact of the new sample design on estimates presented in this report is minimal.
[4]Excludes plans that paid for only one type of service, such as accidents or dental care. A small number of persons were covered by both public and private plans and were included in both categories.

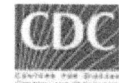

NOTE: Data are based on household interviews of a sample of the civilian noninstitutionalized population.

DATA SOURCE: CDC/NCHS, National Health Interview Survey, 1997–2012, Family Core component.

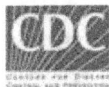

Table 4. Percentage of persons under age 65 who were uninsured at the time of interview, by age group and poverty status: United States, 1997–2012

Age group and year	Poverty status[1]				
	Total	Poor	Near-poor	Not-poor	Unknown
	Percent uninsured[2] (standard error)				
Under 65 years					
1997	17.4 (0.24)	32.7 (0.80)	30.4 (0.70)	8.9 (0.22)	21.6 (0.59)
1998	16.5 (0.26)	32.7 (0.84)	30.8 (0.79)	8.0 (0.22)	20.7 (0.59)
1999	16.0 (0.25)	32.1 (0.93)	30.7 (0.73)	7.8 (0.20)	20.1 (0.48)
2000	16.8 (0.24)	32.7 (0.89)	31.3 (0.69)	8.7 (0.22)	19.7 (0.51)
2001	16.2 (0.26)	31.0 (0.99)	28.6 (0.69)	8.4 (0.21)	20.3 (0.53)
2002	16.5 (0.24)	28.6 (0.80)	28.3 (0.70)	9.5 (0.24)	20.7 (0.55)
2003	17.2 (0.27)	29.4 (0.91)	30.2 (0.70)	9.1 (0.25)	21.3 (0.52)
2004 (Method 1)[3,4]	16.6 (0.23)	30.5 (0.93)	29.1 (0.67)	9.4 (0.23)	18.7 (0.48)
2004 (Method 2)[3,4]	16.4 (0.23)	30.1 (0.91)	28.9 (0.67)	9.4 (0.23)	18.6 (0.48)
2005[3]	16.0 (0.24)	28.4 (0.78)	28.6 (0.63)	9.1 (0.22)	18.5 (0.48)
2006[3,5]	16.8 (0.29)	29.2 (0.98)	30.8 (0.80)	9.7 (0.29)	17.5 (0.49)
2007[6]	16.4 (0.33)	28.0 (1.04)	30.2 (0.91)	9.8 (0.27)	20.8 (0.74)
2008[3]	16.7 (0.36)	27.9 (1.08)	30.6 (0.82)	10.2 (0.27)	21.0 (0.73)
2009[3]	17.5 (0.34)	30.2 (0.89)	29.4 (0.77)	10.7 (0.29)	22.3 (0.85)
2010[3]	18.2 (0.30)	29.5 (0.83)	32.3 (0.69)	10.7 (0.24)	22.7 (0.95)
2011[3,7]	17.3 (0.29)	28.2 (0.66)	30.4 (0.58)	10.1 (0.25)	21.0 (0.64)
2012[3]	16.9 (0.27)	28.3 (0.65)	29.5 (0.56)	9.8 (0.23)	20.4 (0.73)
0–17 years					
1997	13.9 (0.36)	22.4 (0.99)	22.8 (0.96)	6.1 (0.33)	18.3 (0.90)
1998	12.7 (0.34)	21.6 (1.02)	22.5 (0.97)	4.9 (0.29)	16.5 (0.75)
1999	11.8 (0.32)	21.4 (1.13)	21.6 (0.92)	4.4 (0.29)	14.9 (0.69)
2000	12.3 (0.32)	20.6 (1.04)	21.4 (0.93)	5.3 (0.30)	15.0 (0.72)
2001	11.0 (0.34)	18.8 (1.24)	17.0 (0.85)	4.4 (0.26)	15.5 (0.84)
2002	10.5 (0.32)	15.9 (0.97)	15.7 (0.84)	5.3 (0.36)	14.1 (0.76)
2003	10.1 (0.34)	15.4 (1.06)	14.7 (0.88)	4.8 (0.33)	13.5 (0.67)
2004 (Method 1)[3,4]	9.6 (0.29)	16.2 (1.23)	15.5 (0.81)	5.0 (0.30)	10.5 (0.56)
2004 (Method 2)[3,4]	9.4 (0.29)	15.3 (1.17)	15.1 (0.81)	5.0 (0.30)	10.3 (0.56)
2005[3]	8.9 (0.29)	13.0 (0.92)	14.7 (0.79)	4.6 (0.30)	11.0 (0.66)
2006[3,5]	9.3 (0.34)	12.7 (1.06)	16.5 (1.05)	4.8 (0.39)	10.0 (0.63)
2007[6]	8.9 (0.40)	11.4 (1.08)	15.5 (1.10)	4.9 (0.34)	11.8 (1.01)
2008[3]	8.9 (0.43)	12.4 (1.13)	15.6 (1.07)	4.8 (0.39)	11.0 (0.97)
2009[3]	8.2 (0.40)	11.8 (0.94)	12.1 (0.90)	5.0 (0.39)	9.8 (0.99)
2010[3]	7.8 (0.32)	10.2 (0.96)	12.6 (0.73)	4.6 (0.29)	8.8 (0.89)
2011[3,7]	7.0 (0.27)	8.1 (0.62)	11.5 (0.69)	4.0 (0.27)	10.4 (0.76)
2012[3]	6.6 (0.27)	7.5 (0.58)	10.1 (0.70)	4.5 (0.31)	8.2 (0.77)
18–64 years					
1997	18.9 (0.23)	40.2 (0.88)	34.9 (0.71)	9.9 (0.22)	22.9 (0.58)
1998	18.2 (0.27)	40.8 (1.02)	36.0 (0.83)	9.2 (0.23)	22.2 (0.60)
1999	17.8 (0.26)	39.9 (1.11)	36.3 (0.81)	9.0 (0.20)	22.2 (0.50)
2000	18.7 (0.27)	41.1 (1.05)	37.4 (0.77)	10.0 (0.24)	21.5 (0.53)
2001	18.3 (0.27)	39.5 (1.19)	35.6 (0.78)	9.9 (0.22)	22.1 (0.52)
2002	19.1 (0.26)	37.0 (1.09)	36.2 (0.77)	11.0 (0.25)	23.2 (0.56)
2003	20.1 (0.29)	38.2 (1.19)	39.5 (0.81)	10.6 (0.27)	24.2 (0.56)
2004 (Method 1)[3,4]	19.4 (0.26)	40.1 (1.10)	36.9 (0.72)	11.0 (0.26)	21.7 (0.54)
2004 (Method 2)[3,4]	19.3 (0.26)	39.9 (1.09)	36.8 (0.73)	11.0 (0.26)	21.6 (0.54)
2005[3]	18.9 (0.26)	38.5 (0.95)	36.6 (0.73)	10.7 (0.24)	21.2 (0.52)
2006[3,5]	19.8 (0.33)	40.0 (1.33)	38.6 (0.89)	11.4 (0.31)	20.3 (0.54)
2007[6]	19.4 (0.36)	38.6 (1.47)	39.3 (1.01)	11.4 (0.29)	23.8 (0.79)
2008[3]	19.7 (0.40)	37.7 (1.49)	39.9 (0.94)	11.9 (0.28)	24.4 (0.83)
2009[3]	21.1 (0.37)	42.5 (1.20)	39.1 (0.85)	12.5 (0.31)	26.7 (0.99)
2010[3]	22.3 (0.35)	42.2 (0.99)	43.0 (0.74)	12.6 (0.27)	27.1 (1.10)
2011[3,7]	21.3 (0.34)	40.1 (0.92)	40.1 (0.72)	12.0 (0.28)	25.6 (0.77)
2012[3]	20.9 (0.31)	40.1 (0.90)	39.2 (0.68)	11.4 (0.26)	25.7 (0.88)

[1]Based on family income and family size, using the U.S. Census Bureau's poverty thresholds. "Poor" persons are defined as those below the poverty threshold; "Near-poor" persons have incomes of 100% to less than 200% of the poverty threshold; and "Not -poor" persons have incomes of 200% of the poverty threshold or greater. The percentages of respondents with unknown poverty status were 19.1%, 23.6%, 26.4%, 27.0%, 27.1%, 28.1%, 31.5%, 29.6%, 28.9%, 30.7%, 18.0%, 15.8%, 12.3%, 12.2%, 11.5%, and 11.4% in 1997 through 2012. For more information on the "Unknown" income and poverty status categories, see the National Health Interview Survey

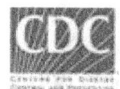

(NHIS) Survey Description document for years 1997–2005, available from: http://www.cdc.gov/nchs/nhis.htm. Estimates may differ from estimates that are based on both reported and imputed income. See Technical Notes for a discussion of the use of imputed income in the stratification of health insurance coverage by poverty status.

[2]A person was defined as uninsured if he or she did not have any private health insurance, Medicare, Medicaid, Children's Health Insurance Program (CHIP), state-sponsored or other government-sponsored health plan, or military plan at the time of the interview. A person was also defined as uninsured if he or she had only Indian Health Service coverage or had only a private plan that paid for one type of service, such as accidents or dental care.

[3]Beginning in the third quarter of 2004, two additional questions were added to the NHIS insurance section to reduce potential errors in reporting Medicare and Medicaid status. Persons aged 65 and over not reporting Medicare coverage were asked explicitly about Medicare coverage, and persons under age 65 with no reported coverage were asked explicitly about Medicaid coverage. Estimates of uninsurance for 2004 were calculated both without the additional information from these questions (noted as Method 1) and with the responses to these questions (noted as Method 2). Respondents who were reclassified as "covered" by the additional questions received the appropriate follow-up questions concerning periods of noncoverage for insured respondents. Beginning in 2005, all estimates were calculated using Method 2. See Technical Notes for additional information.

[4]In 2004, a much larger than expected proportion of respondents reported a family income of "$2." Based on extensive review, these "$2" responses were coded to "not ascertained" for the final 2004 NHIS data files. Effective with the March 2006 Early Release report, the 2004 estimates were recalculated to reflect this editing decision. For a complete discussion, see the NHIS Survey Description document for 2004, available from: http://www.cdc.gov/nchs/nhis.htm. The problem with the "$2" income reports was fixed in the 2005 NHIS.

[5]In 2006, NHIS underwent a sample redesign. The impact of the new sample design on estimates presented in this report is minimal.

[6]In 2007, the income section of NHIS was redesigned, so estimates by poverty status may not be directly comparable with earlier years. See Technical Notes for further information on the income question changes.

[7]In 2011, several new unfolding-bracket income questions were added to the income section of NHIS. See Technical Notes for further information on the income question changes.

NOTE: Data are based on household interviews of a sample of the civilian noninstitutionalized population.

DATA SOURCE: CDC/NCHS, National Health Interview Survey, 1997–2012, Family Core component.

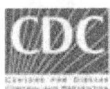

Table 5. Percentage of persons under age 65 with public health plan coverage at the time of interview, by age group and poverty status: United States, 1997–2012

Age group and year	Poverty status[1]				
	Total	Poor	Near-poor	Not-poor	Unknown
	Percent with public health plan coverage[2] (standard error)				
Under 65 years					
1997	13.6 (0.25)	46.1 (1.01)	18.2 (0.56)	5.3 (0.19)	13.2 (0.49)
1998	12.7 (0.26)	44.7 (1.05)	17.5 (0.57)	5.1 (0.23)	13.4 (0.45)
1999	12.4 (0.24)	43.4 (1.04)	20.5 (0.63)	4.8 (0.18)	13.2 (0.43)
2000	12.9 (0.26)	43.7 (1.11)	21.7 (0.62)	5.3 (0.21)	12.8 (0.42)
2001	13.6 (0.26)	45.0 (1.14)	25.0 (0.69)	5.7 (0.21)	13.1 (0.42)
2002	15.2 (0.29)	47.0 (1.07)	27.5 (0.72)	6.1 (0.24)	16.6 (0.45)
2003	16.0 (0.31)	48.8 (1.16)	29.3 (0.75)	6.6 (0.27)	15.8 (0.48)
2004 (Method 1)[3,4]	16.1 (0.29)	50.7 (1.02)	27.6 (0.69)	6.9 (0.23)	16.0 (0.47)
2004 (Method 2)[3,4]	16.2 (0.29)	51.1 (1.01)	27.8 (0.68)	6.9 (0.23)	16.1 (0.47)
2005[3]	16.8 (0.29)	50.6 (0.98)	30.0 (0.72)	7.4 (0.22)	16.4 (0.48)
2006[3,5]	18.1 (0.35)	51.5 (1.17)	30.5 (0.78)	7.5 (0.28)	17.9 (0.64)
2007[6]	18.1 (0.40)	53.3 (1.34)	33.9 (0.91)	7.6 (0.30)	18.6 (0.77)
2008[3]	19.3 (0.42)	55.5 (1.22)	34.7 (0.92)	8.5 (0.30)	19.4 (0.90)
2009[3]	21.0 (0.39)	56.7 (1.06)	36.7 (0.85)	9.0 (0.30)	20.8 (0.88)
2010[3]	22.0 (0.38)	56.0 (0.98)	36.2 (0.63)	9.7 (0.28)	21.0 (0.69)
2011[3,7]	23.0 (0.37)	56.2 (0.82)	37.7 (0.73)	9.9 (0.26)	26.2 (0.95)
2012[3]	23.5 (0.37)	57.1 (0.83)	37.1 (0.66)	10.3 (0.33)	28.8 (0.89)
0–17 years					
1997	21.4 (0.48)	62.1 (1.31)	24.3 (0.93)	6.3 (0.32)	21.4 (0.97)
1998	20.0 (0.49)	61.1 (1.34)	22.9 (0.95)	6.0 (0.39)	22.1 (0.95)
1999	20.4 (0.46)	60.7 (1.37)	28.7 (1.15)	6.0 (0.32)	22.2 (0.88)
2000	22.0 (0.50)	61.8 (1.48)	32.4 (1.13)	7.4 (0.39)	22.1 (0.85)
2001	23.6 (0.50)	65.2 (1.47)	37.0 (1.23)	8.1 (0.39)	23.1 (0.94)
2002	27.1 (0.54)	69.0 (1.33)	42.2 (1.18)	8.9 (0.45)	30.7 (0.99)
2003	28.6 (0.58)	72.3 (1.32)	47.2 (1.27)	9.8 (0.48)	28.5 (1.00)
2004 (Method 1)[3,4]	28.5 (0.54)	72.5 (1.36)	43.4 (1.20)	9.7 (0.45)	30.4 (1.01)
2004 (Method 2)[3,4]	28.7 (0.54)	73.4 (1.34)	43.8 (1.20)	9.7 (0.45)	30.6 (1.01)
2005[3]	29.9 (0.56)	73.3 (1.32)	47.3 (1.21)	10.7 (0.47)	30.8 (1.05)
2006[3,5]	32.3 (0.69)	75.8 (1.32)	49.0 (1.45)	10.4 (0.53)	33.1 (1.25)
2007[6]	32.7 (0.77)	78.7 (1.38)	53.5 (1.44)	11.0 (0.60)	34.0 (1.54)
2008[3]	34.2 (0.79)	79.4 (1.37)	53.4 (1.58)	13.1 (0.62)	35.1 (1.72)
2009[3]	37.7 (0.76)	81.4 (1.11)	58.4 (1.42)	13.7 (0.63)	36.1 (2.05)
2010[3]	39.8 (0.73)	82.0 (1.22)	59.2 (1.16)	14.9 (0.57)	38.1 (1.71)
2011[3,7]	41.0 (0.74)	84.4 (0.87)	60.8 (1.17)	15.0 (0.55)	45.9 (1.70)
2012[3]	42.1 (0.72)	85.9 (0.80)	61.0 (1.30)	15.2 (0.62)	51.8 (1.50)
18–64 years					
1997	10.2 (0.20)	34.3 (0.93)	14.6 (0.51)	5.0 (0.18)	10.1 (0.41)
1998	9.5 (0.21)	32.9 (1.08)	14.1 (0.53)	4.8 (0.21)	10.0 (0.34)
1999	9.0 (0.19)	30.8 (0.98)	15.4 (0.52)	4.4 (0.17)	9.6 (0.33)
2000	9.1 (0.19)	31.1 (1.00)	15.2 (0.54)	4.5 (0.19)	9.1 (0.33)
2001	9.4 (0.21)	30.8 (1.10)	17.8 (0.62)	4.8 (0.20)	9.4 (0.33)
2002	10.3 (0.23)	32.5 (1.10)	18.3 (0.66)	5.1 (0.22)	11.2 (0.35)
2003	10.9 (0.24)	34.0 (1.19)	18.6 (0.68)	5.5 (0.24)	11.1 (0.37)
2004 (Method 1)[3,4]	11.1 (0.22)	36.1 (1.03)	18.5 (0.61)	5.9 (0.21)	10.8 (0.35)
2004 (Method 2)[3,4]	11.1 (0.23)	36.3 (1.03)	18.6 (0.60)	5.9 (0.21)	10.9 (0.35)
2005[3]	11.5 (0.22)	35.6 (0.98)	20.0 (0.61)	6.2 (0.20)	11.3 (0.36)
2006[3,5]	12.4 (0.26)	35.6 (1.25)	20.3 (0.68)	6.5 (0.25)	12.3 (0.48)
2007[6]	12.3 (0.31)	37.0 (1.41)	21.7 (0.85)	6.5 (0.27)	13.4 (0.61)
2008[3]	13.4 (0.33)	40.4 (1.34)	23.1 (0.80)	7.0 (0.28)	14.1 (0.77)
2009[3]	14.4 (0.31)	40.3 (1.21)	24.5 (0.75)	7.6 (0.26)	15.5 (0.69)
2010[3]	15.0 (0.30)	38.8 (0.97)	23.7 (0.55)	8.1 (0.27)	15.6 (0.63)
2011[3,7]	15.9 (0.29)	39.6 (0.93)	25.9 (0.69)	8.3 (0.23)	17.6 (0.73)
2012[3]	16.4 (0.29)	40.8 (0.94)	25.2 (0.57)	8.7 (0.29)	18.9 (0.76)

[1]Based on family income and family size, using the U.S. Census Bureau's poverty thresholds. "Poor" persons are defined as those below the poverty threshold; "Near-poor" persons have incomes of 100% to less than 200% of the poverty threshold; and "Not-poor" persons have incomes of 200% of the poverty threshold or greater. The percentages of respondents with unknown poverty status were 119.1%, 23.6%, 26.4%, 27.0%, 27.1%, 28.1%, 31.5%, 29.6%, 28.9%, 30.7%, 18.0%, 15.8%, 12.3%, 12.2%, 11.5%, and 11.4% in

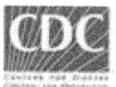

1997 through 2012. For more information on the "Unknown" income and poverty status categories, see the National Health Interview Survey (*NHIS*) *Survey Description* document for years 1997–2005, available from: http://www.cdc.gov/nchs/nhis.htm. Estimates may differ from estimates that are based on both reported and imputed income. See Technical Notes for a discussion of the use of imputed income in the stratification of health insurance coverage by poverty status.

[2]The category "Public health plan coverage" includes Medicaid, Children's Health Insurance Program (CHIP), state-sponsored or other government-sponsored health plans, Medicare (disability), and military plans. A small number of persons were covered by both public and private plans and were included in both categories. See Table 6 for persons covered by private plans.

[3]Beginning in the third quarter of 2004, two additional questions were added to the NHIS insurance section to reduce potential errors in reporting Medicare and Medicaid status. Persons aged 65 and over not reporting Medicare coverage were asked explicitly about Medicare coverage, and persons under age 65 with no reported coverage were asked explicitly about Medicaid coverage. Estimates of uninsurance for 2004 were calculated both without the additional information from these questions (noted as Method 1) and with the responses to these questions (noted as Method 2). Respondents who were reclassified as "covered" by the additional questions received the appropriate follow-up questions concerning periods of noncoverage for insured respondents. Beginning in 2005, all estimates were calculated using Method 2. See Technical Notes for additional information.

[4]In 2004, a much larger than expected proportion of respondents reported a family income of "$2." Based on extensive review, these "$2" responses were coded to "not ascertained" for the final 2004 NHIS data files. Effective with the March 2006 Early Release report, the 2004 estimates were recalculated to reflect this editing decision. For a complete discussion, see the *NHIS Survey Description* document for 2004, available from: http://www.cdc.gov/nchs/nhis.htm. The problem with the "$2" income reports was fixed in the 2005 NHIS.

[5]In 2006, NHIS underwent a sample redesign. The impact of the new sample design on estimates presented in this report is minimal.

[6]In 2007, the income section of NHIS was redesigned, and estimates by poverty status may not be directly comparable with earlier years. See Technical Notes for further information on the income question changes.

[7]In 2011, several new unfolding-bracket income questions were added to the income section of NHIS. See Technical Notes for further information on the income question changes.

NOTE: Data are based on household interviews of a sample of the civilian noninstitutionalized population.

DATA SOURCE: CDC/NCHS, National Health Interview Survey, 1997–2012, Family Core component.

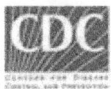

Table 6. Percentage of persons under age 65 with private health insurance coverage at the time of interview, by age group and poverty status: United States, 1997–2012

Age group and year	Poverty status[1]				
	Total	Poor	Near-poor	Not-poor	Unknown
	Percent with private health insurance coverage[2] (standard error)				
Under 65 years					
1997	70.8 (0.35)	22.9 (0.93)	53.5 (0.80)	87.6 (0.27)	66.7 (0.71)
1998	72.0 (0.36)	23.1 (1.02)	53.0 (0.92)	88.1 (0.29)	67.1 (0.71)
1999	73.1 (0.36)	26.1 (1.12)	50.9 (0.86)	88.9 (0.24)	68.0 (0.65)
2000	71.8 (0.34)	25.2 (1.00)	49.1 (0.87)	87.4 (0.28)	68.8 (0.63)
2001	71.6 (0.37)	25.5 (1.13)	48.4 (0.85)	87.2 (0.27)	67.8 (0.69)
2002	69.8 (0.39)	26.0 (1.14)	46.5 (0.89)	86.0 (0.33)	63.9 (0.71)
2003	68.2 (0.40)	23.4 (1.21)	42.3 (0.90)	85.8 (0.34)	64.1 (0.68)
2004[3]	68.6 (0.39)	20.0 (1.11)	44.9 (0.85)	85.0 (0.32)	66.3 (0.70)
2005	68.4 (0.39)	22.1 (0.89)	43.2 (0.89)	84.7 (0.30)	66.2 (0.68)
2006[4]	66.5 (0.48)	20.6 (1.29)	40.6 (0.91)	84.1 (0.41)	65.7 (0.79)
2007[5]	66.8 (0.53)	20.1 (1.41)	37.9 (1.00)	83.8 (0.40)	61.7 (1.04)
2008[3]	65.4 (0.58)	17.9 (1.21)	36.3 (1.00)	82.5 (0.38)	60.7 (1.16)
2009[3]	62.9 (0.54)	14.1 (0.87)	35.9 (0.93)	81.6 (0.42)	57.9 (1.24)
2010[3]	61.2 (0.50)	15.5 (0.70)	33.2 (0.77)	81.0 (0.36)	57.3 (1.08)
2011[3,6]	61.2 (0.51)	16.6 (0.77)	33.5 (0.75)	81.4 (0.36)	53.9 (1.09)
2012[3]	61.0 (0.47)	16.1 (0.83)	35.2 (0.75)	81.3 (0.39)	52.1 (1.00)
0–17 years					
1997	66.2 (0.57)	17.5 (1.09)	55.0 (1.15)	88.9 (0.43)	61.7 (1.18)
1998	68.5 (0.55)	19.3 (1.17)	56.3 (1.22)	89.9 (0.48)	62.1 (1.13)
1999	69.1 (0.55)	20.2 (1.16)	52.1 (1.23)	90.6 (0.39)	63.8 (1.02)
2000	67.1 (0.53)	19.5 (1.21)	48.8 (1.23)	88.4 (0.47)	64.2 (0.99)
2001	66.7 (0.57)	18.1 (1.12)	48.4 (1.23)	88.4 (0.40)	62.2 (1.16)
2002	63.9 (0.61)	17.2 (1.08)	44.9 (1.29)	86.9 (0.54)	56.3 (1.19)
2003	62.6 (0.60)	14.4 (1.06)	39.9 (1.28)	86.5 (0.56)	58.8 (1.07)
2004[3]	63.1 (0.59)	12.6 (0.97)	43.0 (1.29)	86.4 (0.52)	60.0 (1.11)
2005	62.4 (0.60)	15.0 (1.10)	40.0 (1.31)	85.6 (0.52)	59.3 (1.16)
2006[4]	59.7 (0.72)	13.1 (1.10)	36.9 (1.37)	85.9 (0.63)	57.8 (1.28)
2007[5]	59.9 (0.82)	11.9 (1.08)	34.0 (1.46)	85.1 (0.63)	54.8 (1.82)
2008[3]	58.3 (0.84)	10.4 (0.95)	32.9 (1.46)	83.1 (0.67)	54.8 (1.78)
2009[3]	55.7 (0.86)	8.2 (0.81)	32.8 (1.43)	82.4 (0.73)	55.3 (2.07)
2010[3]	53.8 (0.75)	9.2 (0.70)	30.5 (1.18)	81.4 (0.61)	53.7 (1.74)
2011[3,6]	53.3 (0.76)	8.9 (0.72)	29.9 (1.07)	82.1 (0.58)	44.5 (1.66)
2012[3]	52.8 (0.73)	8.8 (0.78)	31.1 (1.18)	81.3 (0.64)	41.2 (1.49)
18–64 years					
1997	72.8 (0.30)	26.8 (1.09)	52.6 (0.76)	87.1 (0.26)	68.6 (0.65)
1998	73.5 (0.32)	25.8 (1.17)	50.9 (0.90)	87.4 (0.27)	69.1 (0.66)
1999	74.7 (0.33)	30.4 (1.39)	50.2 (0.85)	88.2 (0.24)	69.7 (0.60)
2000	73.8 (0.32)	29.2 (1.16)	49.3 (0.83)	87.1 (0.27)	70.6 (0.61)
2001	73.7 (0.33)	31.7 (1.41)	48.4 (0.82)	86.8 (0.28)	69.9 (0.61)
2002	72.3 (0.35)	31.8 (1.50)	47.5 (0.85)	85.7 (0.30)	66.9 (0.62)
2003	70.6 (0.36)	29.0 (1.60)	43.7 (0.88)	85.5 (0.33)	66.0 (0.62)
2004[3]	70.9 (0.36)	24.9 (1.39)	46.0 (0.79)	84.6 (0.31)	68.6 (0.65)
2005	70.9 (0.36)	26.8 (1.03)	45.0 (0.85)	84.4 (0.29)	68.7 (0.61)
2006[4]	69.2 (0.43)	25.5 (1.72)	42.6 (0.92)	83.6 (0.40)	68.6 (0.71)
2007[5]	69.6 (0.47)	25.4 (1.92)	40.4 (1.01)	83.4 (0.38)	64.0 (0.92)
2008[3]	68.1 (0.54)	22.7 (1.65)	38.3 (1.01)	82.4 (0.37)	62.7 (1.13)
2009[3]	65.8 (0.47)	18.0 (1.15)	37.7 (0.84)	81.4 (0.38)	58.8 (1.13)
2010[3]	64.1 (0.46)	19.6 (0.89)	34.7 (0.74)	80.8 (0.36)	58.4 (1.11)
2011[3,6]	64.2 (0.45)	21.2 (1.02)	35.4 (0.75)	81.1 (0.35)	58.1 (0.96)
2012[3]	64.1 (0.42)	20.2 (1.09)	37.2 (0.74)	81.3 (0.38)	56.9 (0.92)

[1]Based on family income and family size, using the U.S. Census Bureau's poverty thresholds. "Poor" persons are defined as those below the poverty threshold; "Near-poor" persons have incomes of 100% to less than 200% of the poverty threshold; and "Not-poor" persons have incomes of 200% of the poverty threshold or greater. The percentages of respondents with unknown poverty status were 19.1%, 23.6%, 26.4%, 27.0%, 27.1%, 28.1%, 31.5%, 29.6%, 28.9%, 30.7%, 18.0%, 15.8%, 12.3%, 12.2%, 11.5%, and 11.4% in 1997 through 2012. For more information on the "Unknown" income and poverty status categories, see the National Health Interview Survey (*NHIS*) *Survey Description* document for years 1997–2005, available from: http://www.cdc.gov/nchs/nhis.htm. Estimates may differ

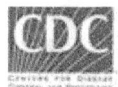

from estimates that are based on both reported and imputed income. See Technical Notes for a discussion of the use of imputed income in the stratification of health insurance coverage by poverty status.

[2]The category "Private health insurance" excludes plans that paid for only one type of service, such as accidents or dental care. A small number of persons were covered by both public and private plans and thus were included in both categories. See Table 5 for persons covered by public plans.

[3]In 2004, a much larger than expected proportion of respondents reported a family income of "$2." Based on extensive review, these "$2" responses were coded to "not ascertained" for the final 2004 NHIS data files. Effective with the March 2006 Early Release report the 2004 estimates were recalculated to reflect this editing decision. For a complete discussion, see the *NHIS Survey Description* document for 2004, available from: http://www.cdc.gov/nchs/nhis.htm. The problem with the "$2" income reports was fixed in the 2005 NHIS.

[4]In 2006, NHIS underwent a sample redesign. The impact of the new sample design on estimates presented in this report is minimal.

[5]In 2007, the income section of NHIS was redesigned, and estimates by poverty status may not be directly comparable with earlier years. See Technical Notes for further information on the income question changes.

[6]In 2011, several new unfolding-bracket income questions were added to the income section of NHIS. See Technical Notes for further information on the income question changes.

NOTE: Data are based on household interviews of a sample of the civilian noninstitutionalized population.

DATA SOURCE: CDC/NCHS, National Health Interview Survey, 1997–2012, Family Core component.

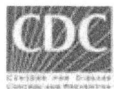

Table 7. Percentages of persons who lacked health insurance coverage at the time of interview, for at least part of the past year, and for more than a year, by selected demographic characteristics: United States, 2012

Selected characteristic	Uninsured[1] at the time of interview	Uninsured[1] for at least part of the past year[2]	Uninsured[1] for more than a year[2]
	Percent (standard error)		
Age			
All ages	14.7 (0.23)	18.6 (0.27)	11.1 (0.22)
Under 65 years	16.9 (0.27)	21.3 (0.31)	12.7 (0.24)
0–17 years	6.6 (0.27)	10.4 (0.35)	3.7 (0.19)
18–64 years	20.9 (0.31)	25.5 (0.34)	16.2 (0.29)
18–24 years	24.6 (0.67)	30.8 (0.69)	17.9 (0.58)
25–34 years	28.2 (0.54)	34.8 (0.61)	21.5 (0.51)
35–44 years	21.6 (0.52)	26.2 (0.55)	17.1 (0.47)
45–64 years	15.6 (0.32)	18.6 (0.35)	12.5 (0.30)
65 years and over	0.9 (0.09)	1.6 (0.12)	0.7 (0.08)
0–18 years	7.0 (0.27)	10.8 (0.35)	3.9 (0.19)
19–25 years	26.4 (0.72)	33.0 (0.72)	19.6 (0.62)
Sex			
Male:			
All ages	16.3 (0.28)	19.9 (0.31)	12.7 (0.26)
Under 65 years	18.5 (0.31)	22.4 (0.34)	14.3 (0.29)
0–17 years	6.5 (0.29)	10.2 (0.39)	3.6 (0.21)
18–64 years	23.2 (0.38)	27.3 (0.39)	18.6 (0.36)
18–24 years	27.7 (0.91)	32.5 (0.92)	21.3 (0.83)
25–34 years	32.8 (0.69)	38.6 (0.75)	26.4 (0.66)
35–44 years	24.1 (0.68)	28.4 (0.71)	19.7 (0.60)
45–64 years	16.3 (0.39)	19.1 (0.42)	13.2 (0.37)
65 years and over	1.1 (0.15)	2.0 (0.18)	1.0 (0.14)
0–18 years	6.9 (0.29)	10.7 (0.39)	3.9 (0.21)
19–25 years	30.3 (1.01)	35.2 (0.97)	23.8 (0.90)
Female:			
All ages	13.2 (0.25)	17.4 (0.30)	9.5 (0.22)
Under 65 years	15.4 (0.29)	20.2 (0.34)	11.1 (0.25)
0–17 years	6.8 (0.36)	10.6 (0.43)	3.7 (0.24)
18–64 years	18.6 (0.33)	23.7 (0.37)	13.8 (0.30)
18–24 years	21.4 (0.73)	29.2 (0.84)	14.5 (0.60)
25–34 years	23.7 (0.62)	31.1 (0.74)	16.8 (0.56)
35–44 years	19.2 (0.53)	24.0 (0.59)	14.6 (0.51)
45–64 years	14.9 (0.37)	18.1 (0.40)	11.8 (0.33)
65 years and over	0.7 (0.09)	1.4 (0.14)	0.5 (0.08)
0–18 years	7.1 (0.35)	11.0 (0.43)	3.9 (0.24)
19–25 years	22.6 (0.76)	30.9 (0.85)	15.5 (0.62)
Race/ethnicity			
Hispanic or Latino	28.9 (0.68)	33.2 (0.64)	23.9 (0.65)
Non-Hispanic:			
White, single race	10.6 (0.23)	14.3 (0.29)	7.6 (0.19)
Black, single race	16.3 (0.46)	20.5 (0.53)	11.6 (0.41)
Asian, single race	14.9 (0.87)	18.2 (0.96)	11.5 (0.72)
Other races and multiple races	15.5 (1.25)	21.3 (1.31)	9.1 (0.76)
Region			
Northeast	10.0 (0.49)	13.3 (0.66)	7.1 (0.51)
Midwest	11.8 (0.42)	15.7 (0.53)	8.6 (0.31)
South	17.5 (0.44)	21.4 (0.50)	13.5 (0.41)
West	16.8 (0.42)	21.0 (0.45)	12.6 (0.40)
Education[3]			
Less than high school	32.1 (0.72)	36.0 (0.73)	27.5 (0.72)
High school diploma or GED[4]	21.5 (0.40)	25.3 (0.43)	16.9 (0.38)
More than high school	11.6 (0.23)	15.6 (0.27)	8.3 (0.19)

See footnotes at end of table.

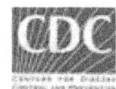

Table 7. Percentages of persons who lacked health insurance coverage at the time of interview, for at least part of the past year, and for more than a year, by selected demographic characteristics: United States, 2012 (cont.)

Selected characteristic	Uninsured[1] at the time of interview	Uninsured[1] for at least part of the past year[2]	Uninsured[1] for more than a year[2]
	Percent (standard error)		
Employment status[5]			
Employed	18.5 (0.32)	22.9 (0.35)	14.8 (0.31)
Unemployed	47.1 (0.88)	54.2 (0.85)	33.3 (0.89)
Not in workforce	20.1 (0.44)	24.6 (0.48)	15.3 (0.39)
Marital status[3]			
Married	12.6 (0.29)	15.6 (0.32)	9.8 (0.27)
Widowed	5.0 (0.36)	6.2 (0.39)	3.9 (0.33)
Divorced or separated	21.0 (0.51)	26.0 (0.55)	16.4 (0.47)
Living with partner	32.4 (0.87)	39.6 (0.84)	25.3 (0.81)
Never married	25.6 (0.46)	30.8 (0.50)	19.6 (0.41)

[1]A person was defined as uninsured if he or she did not have any private health insurance, Medicare, Medicaid, Children's Health Insurance Program (CHIP), state-sponsored or other government-sponsored health plan, or military plan. A person was also defined as uninsured if he or she had only Indian Health Service coverage or had only a private plan that paid for one type of service, such as accidents or dental care.
[2]A year is defined as the 12 months prior to interview.
[3]Shown only for persons aged 18 and over.
[4]GED is General Educational Development high school equivalency diploma.
[5]Shown only for persons aged 18–64.

NOTE: Data are based on household interviews of a sample of the civilian noninstitutionalized population.

DATA SOURCE: CDC/NCHS, National Health Interview Survey, 2012, Family Core component.

(Released 06/2013)

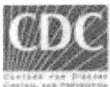

Table 8. Percentages of persons aged 19–25 and 26–35 who were uninsured, had private health insurance coverage, and had public health plan coverage at the time of interview, by year and quarter: United States, January 2008–December 2012

Year and quarter (Q)	Persons aged 19–25			Persons aged 26–35		
	Uninsured[1]	Private health insurance coverage[2]	Public health plan coverage[3]	Uninsured[1]	Private health insurance coverage[2]	Public health plan coverage[3]
	Percent (standard error)					
2008 full year	30.9 (0.87)	55.7 (1.02)	14.0 (0.75)	25.5 (0.64)	63.7 (0.77)	11.3 (0.48)
Q1	29.4 (1.65)	58.5 (1.95)	13.0 (1.62)	25.8 (1.16)	62.9 (1.49)	11.7 (0.90)
Q2	30.4 (1.25)	56.6 (1.49)	13.9 (0.94)	24.8 (1.13)	64.1 (1.30)	11.8 (0.89)
Q3	31.9 (1.34)	54.8 (1.53)	13.8 (0.90)	24.6 (1.05)	64.6 (1.19)	11.6 (0.72)
Q4	32.1 (2.19)	52.9 (2.46)	15.5 (1.60)	27.0 (1.55)	63.3 (1.71)	10.1 (0.98)
2009 full year	32.7 (0.82)	52.6 (0.91)	15.0 (0.62)	26.5 (0.70)	61.3 (0.82)	12.8 (0.45)
Q1	30.2 (2.02)	56.3 (2.25)	13.6 (1.53)	25.3 (1.99)	63.7 (2.15)	11.8 (1.25)
Q2	33.5 (1.30)	52.0 (1.51)	14.7 (0.98)	26.5 (1.11)	62.5 (1.28)	11.6 (0.80)
Q3	35.1 (1.36)	50.2 (1.50)	14.9 (1.05)	27.4 (1.10)	60.2 (1.38)	12.7 (0.84)
Q4	32.2 (1.03)	51.7 (1.36)	16.7 (0.95)	26.9 (0.92)	58.7 (1.11)	15.0 (0.70)
2010 full year	33.9 (0.73)	51.0 (0.84)	15.7 (0.55)	27.5 (0.62)	59.5 (0.74)	13.5 (0.45)
Q1	33.8 (1.47)	50.0 (1.69)	16.8 (1.15)	27.6 (1.17)	60.3 (1.35)	12.6 (0.81)
Q2	34.8 (1.40)	51.5 (1.57)	13.8 (0.94)	27.9 (1.27)	59.7 (1.38)	13.1 (0.73)
Q3	35.6 (1.39)	49.3 (1.50)	15.8 (1.11)	27.7 (1.14)	59.5 (1.22)	13.5 (0.79)
Q4	31.2 (1.33)	53.3 (1.57)	16.3 (1.08)	27.0 (1.17)	58.5 (1.32)	15.0 (0.88)
2011 full year	27.9 (0.71)	56.3 (0.85)	16.8 (0.60)	27.7 (0.59)	58.8 (0.69)	14.1 (0.39)
Q1	30.4 (1.33)	53.2 (1.69)	16.9 (1.12)	26.0 (1.12)	59.9 (1.27)	14.7 (0.82)
Q2	27.3 (1.36)	58.4 (1.62)	15.2 (0.91)	28.3 (1.06)	58.6 (1.28)	13.8 (0.73)
Q3	28.4 (1.37)	54.7 (1.57)	17.8 (1.17)	28.4 (1.07)	58.3 (1.14)	13.9 (0.74)
Q4	25.2 (1.24)	58.8 (1.46)	17.1 (0.98)	28.2 (1.17)	58.3 (1.38)	14.0 (0.77)
2012 full year	26.4 (0.72)	57.2 (0.85)	17.5 (0.59)	27.7 (0.53)	58.7 (0.67)	14.2 (0.43)
Q1	27.5 (1.41)	55.1 (1.74)	18.2 (1.13)	29.1 (1.13)	57.9 (1.17)	13.6 (0.74)
Q2	24.9 (1.37)	59.2 (1.93)	17.2 (1.03)	25.1 (1.03)	60.9 (1.32)	14.5 (0.87)
Q3	26.3 (1.24)	56.7 (1.59)	17.9 (1.24)	28.7 (1.19)	57.0 (1.33)	14.8 (0.80)
Q4	27.0 (1.41)	57.9 (1.63)	16.4 (1.00)	27.7 (0.95)	58.8 (1.26)	14.1 (0.81)

[1]A person was defined as uninsured if he or she did not have any private health insurance, Medicare, Medicaid, Children's Health Insurance Program (CHIP), state-sponsored or other government-sponsored health plan, or military plan. A person was also defined as uninsured if he or she had only Indian Health Service coverage or had only a private plan that paid for one type of service, such as accidents or dental care.
[2]Excludes plans that paid for only one type of service, such as accidents or dental care.
[3]Includes Medicaid, CHIP, state-sponsored or other government-sponsored health plan, Medicare (disability), and military plans.

NOTE: Data are based on household interviews of a sample of the civilian noninstitutionalized population.

DATA SOURCE: CDC/NCHS, National Health Interview Survey, 2008–2012, Family Core component.

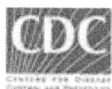

Table 9. Percentages of persons aged 19–25 who were uninsured, had private health insurance coverage, and had public health plan coverage at the time of interview, by year, quarter, and sex: United States, January 2008–December 2012

Year and quarter (Q)	Males			Females		
	Uninsured[1]	Private health insurance coverage[2]	Public health plan coverage[3]	Uninsured[1]	Private health insurance coverage[2]	Public health plan coverage[3]
	Percent (standard error)					
2008 full year	35.2 (1.18)	56.2 (1.23)	9.3 (0.82)	26.7 (1.05)	55.2 (1.25)	18.7 (0.95)
Q1	32.9 (2.38)	59.2 (2.40)	9.1 (2.11)	25.8 (1.67)	57.7 (2.23)	16.8 (1.62)
Q2	35.8 (1.91)	55.3 (2.10)	9.6 (1.13)	25.1 (1.54)	57.9 (1.82)	18.1 (1.34)
Q3	35.1 (2.15)	56.2 (2.11)	8.9 (1.00)	28.7 (1.83)	53.4 (1.89)	18.7 (1.44)
Q4	37.0 (2.99)	54.0 (3.04)	9.7 (1.55)	27.3 (2.38)	51.9 (2.90)	21.1 (2.43)
2009 full year	37.7 (1.15)	52.3 (1.18)	10.3 (0.66)	27.7 (0.89)	52.9 (1.10)	19.7 (0.91)
Q1	34.9 (2.98)	55.6 (2.91)	9.8 (1.65)	25.6 (2.13)	57.1 (2.65)	17.4 (2.16)
Q2	40.2 (1.81)	49.8 (1.93)	10.3 (1.16)	26.8 (1.54)	54.3 (1.91)	19.0 (1.39)
Q3	39.6 (1.83)	51.2 (1.90)	9.2 (1.09)	30.6 (1.67)	49.2 (1.95)	20.8 (1.54)
Q4	36.2 (1.65)	52.6 (1.71)	11.7 (0.92)	28.2 (1.32)	50.9 (1.80)	21.6 (1.39)
2010 full year	39.2 (0.99)	51.2 (1.04)	10.0 (0.53)	28.4 (0.82)	50.9 (1.01)	21.5 (0.84)
Q1	40.0 (2.01)	50.2 (2.10)	10.3 (1.03)	27.7 (1.77)	49.8 (2.07)	23.2 (1.70)
Q2	40.7 (1.81)	49.9 (1.89)	9.4 (1.04)	28.9 (1.67)	53.1 (1.89)	18.2 (1.30)
Q3	42.1 (2.03)	48.1 (2.06)	10.4 (1.09)	28.8 (1.50)	50.6 (1.85)	21.3 (1.72)
Q4	34.0 (1.74)	56.5 (1.90)	9.8 (1.01)	28.3 (1.61)	50.1 (1.98)	23.2 (1.67)
2011 full year	30.7 (0.92)	57.5 (1.01)	12.6 (0.61)	25.0 (0.84)	54.9 (1.03)	21.1 (0.81)
Q1	33.3 (1.77)	53.9 (2.10)	12.9 (1.32)	27.5 (1.51)	52.5 (1.94)	21.0 (1.54)
Q2	31.1 (2.04)	59.6 (2.26)	10.0 (0.98)	23.5 (1.48)	57.2 (1.72)	20.3 (1.31)
Q3	30.3 (1.71)	57.1 (1.82)	13.8 (1.26)	26.5 (1.66)	52.2 (1.96)	21.9 (1.54)
Q4	28.0 (1.58)	59.5 (1.76)	13.4 (1.16)	22.5 (1.58)	58.1 (1.93)	20.8 (1.34)
2012 full year	30.3 (1.01)	58.2 (1.02)	12.3 (0.62)	22.6 (0.76)	56.2 (1.03)	22.6 (0.78)
Q1	32.3 (1.94)	56.6 (2.15)	12.0 (1.09)	22.9 (1.61)	53.7 (2.06)	24.4 (1.60)
Q2	28.2 (1.74)	59.4 (2.10)	13.7 (1.18)	21.6 (1.68)	59.1 (2.38)	20.8 (1.43)
Q3	29.8 (1.75)	57.9 (2.01)	12.6 (1.47)	22.8 (1.39)	55.5 (1.81)	23.2 (1.55)
Q4	30.9 (1.88)	58.9 (2.05)	10.9 (1.05)	23.1 (1.51)	57.0 (1.98)	21.8 (1.49)

[1]A person was defined as uninsured if he or she did not have any private health insurance, Medicare, Medicaid, Children's Health Insurance Program (CHIP), state-sponsored or other government-sponsored health plan, or military plan. A person was also defined as uninsured if he or she had only Indian Health Service coverage or had only a private plan that paid for one type of service, such as accidents or dental care.
[2]Excludes plans that paid for only one type of service, such as accidents or dental care.
[3]Includes Medicaid, CHIP, state-sponsored or other government-sponsored health plan, Medicare (disability), and military plans.

NOTE: Data are based on household interviews of a sample of the civilian noninstitutionalized population.

DATA SOURCE: CDC/NCHS, National Health Interview Survey, 2008–2012, Family Core component.

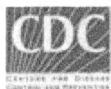

Table 10. Percentages of persons aged 19–25 who were uninsured, had private health insurance coverage, and had public health plan coverage at the time of interview, by year, quarter, and region: United States, January 2010–December 2012

Year, quarter (Q), and region	Uninsured[1]	Private health insurance coverage[2]	Public health plan coverage[3]
	Percent (standard error)		
Total 2010	33.9 (0.73)	51.0 (0.84)	15.7 (0.55)
Q1	33.8 (1.47)	50.0 (1.69)	16.8 (1.15)
Q2	34.8 (1.40)	51.5 (1.57)	13.8 (0.94)
Q3	35.6 (1.39)	49.3 (1.50)	15.8 (1.11)
Q4	31.2 (1.33)	53.3 (1.57)	16.3 (1.08)
Total 2011	27.9 (0.71)	56.3 (0.85)	16.8 (0.60)
Q1	30.4 (1.33)	53.2 (1.69)	16.9 (1.12)
Q2	27.3 (1.36)	58.4 (1.62)	15.2 (0.91)
Q3	28.4 (1.37)	54.7 (1.57)	17.8 (1.17)
Q4	25.2 (1.24)	58.8 (1.46)	17.1 (0.98)
Total 2012	26.4 (0.72)	57.2 (0.85)	17.5 (0.59)
Q1	27.5 (1.41)	55.1 (1.74)	18.2 (1.13)
Q2	24.9 (1.37)	59.2 (1.93)	17.2 (1.03)
Q3	26.3 (1.24)	56.7 (1.59)	17.9 (1.24)
Q4	27.0 (1.41)	57.9 (1.63)	16.4 (1.00)
Northeast 2010	25.6 (1.74)	54.6 (2.12)	20.4 (1.41)
Q1	23.7 (2.48)	55.4 (3.97)	21.8 (3.46)
Q2	28.1 (2.67)	53.5 (4.06)	18.5 (3.18)
Q3	24.2 (3.65)	54.3 (3.39)	22.6 (3.20)
Q4	26.3 (3.32)	55.4 (2.73)	18.9 (2.87)
Northeast 2011	20.4 (1.35)	61.0 (2.17)	19.1 (1.73)
Q1	28.6 (3.54)	50.4 (4.02)	21.0 (3.11)
Q2	18.9 (3.10)	64.9 (4.26)	16.9 (2.19)
Q3	15.7 (2.24)	64.5 (3.70)	19.9 (3.20)
Q4	19.2 (2.92)	63.9 (2.74)	18.0 (2.61)
Northeast 2012	18.2 (1.47)	62.6 (1.42)	20.0 (1.37)
Q1	19.8 (2.30)	60.9 (3.87)	20.1 (3.22)
Q2	19.2 (2.94)	64.0 (4.84)	17.2 (2.66)
Q3	13.8 (2.31)	62.9 (4.53)	24.6 (3.92)
Q4	19.4 (2.87)	64.1 (3.57)	17.2 (2.37)
Midwest 2010	28.6 (1.36)	56.3 (1.78)	16.0 (1.22)
Q1	30.3 (2.77)	53.7 (3.37)	16.7 (2.46)
Q2	30.2 (2.88)	55.1 (3.19)	15.1 (1.98)
Q3	29.3 (2.80)	55.9 (3.11)	15.6 (2.47)
Q4	24.5 (2.85)	60.5 (3.75)	16.9 (2.48)
Midwest 2011	21.9 (1.40)	62.9 (1.58)	16.1 (1.11)
Q1	21.8 (2.42)	62.0 (3.25)	17.0 (2.40)
Q2	20.4 (2.27)	67.7 (2.72)	12.4 (1.89)
Q3	25.4 (3.50)	56.1 (3.54)	19.5 (2.59)
Q4	19.8 (2.21)	66.1 (2.91)	15.1 (2.05)
Midwest 2012	21.8 (1.12)	63.4 (1.59)	16.3 (1.20)
Q1	21.5 (2.62)	60.8 (4.08)	19.1 (2.88)
Q2	20.0 (2.94)	67.4 (4.19)	15.3 (1.98)
Q3	22.6 (2.18)	61.3 (3.28)	16.9 (2.69)
Q4	23.8 (2.88)	63.6 (3.24)	13.5 (1.72)

See footnotes at end of table.

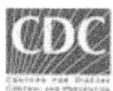

Table 10. Percentages of persons aged 19–25 who were uninsured, had private health insurance coverage, and had public health plan coverage at the time of interview, by year, quarter, and region: United States, January 2010–December 2012 (cont.)

Year, quarter (Q), and region	Uninsured[1]	Private health insurance coverage[2]	Public health plan coverage[3]
		Percent (standard error)	
South 2010	39.3 (1.41)	47.8 (1.47)	13.3 (0.77)
Q1	37.8 (2.57)	48.0 (2.95)	14.7 (1.57)
Q2	41.7 (2.68)	46.3 (2.73)	12.0 (1.45)
Q3	44.4 (2.43)	45.2 (2.36)	10.9 (1.32)
Q4	33.8 (2.29)	51.6 (2.61)	15.3 (1.49)
South 2011	33.9 (1.39)	51.1 (1.37)	16.0 (1.02)
Q1	34.4 (2.32)	50.1 (2.69)	16.1 (1.65)
Q2	36.3 (2.34)	49.4 (2.24)	15.3 (1.60)
Q3	34.8 (2.14)	50.4 (2.36)	16.3 (1.92)
Q4	29.8 (2.32)	55.1 (2.53)	16.3 (1.66)
South 2012	31.2 (1.35)	53.0 (1.53)	16.9 (0.95)
Q1	32.6 (2.72)	49.7 (2.83)	18.5 (1.66)
Q2	29.3 (2.19)	54.5 (2.85)	17.6 (1.74)
Q3	32.6 (2.14)	52.2 (2.42)	15.9 (1.48)
Q4	30.4 (2.53)	55.6 (2.75)	15.7 (1.64)
West 2010	36.2 (1.26)	48.5 (1.53)	15.6 (1.25)
Q1	38.2 (3.15)	45.5 (3.11)	16.7 (2.46)
Q2	34.0 (2.61)	53.9 (2.87)	12.1 (1.35)
Q3	36.3 (2.47)	46.0 (3.31)	18.3 (2.46)
Q4	36.9 (2.35)	48.0 (3.33)	15.6 (2.27)
West 2011	30.1 (1.30)	53.8 (1.89)	17.0 (1.19)
Q1	33.4 (2.61)	51.5 (3.97)	15.8 (2.36)
Q2	28.0 (2.36)	57.2 (3.31)	15.9 (1.71)
Q3	31.0 (2.89)	52.6 (3.54)	16.8 (1.87)
Q4	28.4 (2.32)	53.2 (3.12)	19.5 (1.77)
West 2012	29.7 (1.72)	53.5 (2.02)	17.7 (1.37)
Q1	31.4 (2.68)	53.9 (3.08)	15.6 (1.73)
Q2	27.9 (2.68)	54.4 (3.77)	18.6 (2.15)
Q3	29.6 (3.04)	54.4 (3.20)	17.0 (2.73)
Q4	29.9 (2.86)	51.6 (3.58)	19.8 (2.48)

[1]A person was defined as uninsured if he or she did not have any private health insurance, Medicare, Medicaid, Children's Health Insurance Program (CHIP), state-sponsored or other government-sponsored health plan, or military plan. A person was also defined as uninsured if he or she had only Indian Health Service coverage or had only a private plan that paid for one type of service, such as accidents or dental care.

[2]Excludes plans that paid for only one type of service, such as accidents or dental care.

[3]Includes Medicaid, CHIP, state-sponsored or other government-sponsored health plan, Medicare (disability), and military plans.

NOTE: Data are based on household interviews of a sample of the civilian noninstitutionalized population.

DATA SOURCE: CDC/NCHS, National Health Interview Survey, 2010–2012, Family Core component.

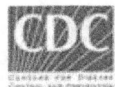

Table 11. Percentages of persons aged 19–25 who were uninsured, had private health insurance coverage, and had public health plan coverage at the time of interview, by race/ethnicity, year, and quarter: United States, January 2008–December 2012

Race/ethnicity, year, and quarter (Q)	Uninsured[1]	Private health insurance coverage[2]	Public health plan coverage[3]
		Percent (standard error)	
Hispanic			
2008	53.4 (1.72)	31.2 (1.49)	15.7 (1.27)
Q1	50.9 (3.12)	34.9 (2.82)	14.4 (1.77)
Q2	51.9 (2.91)	34.2 (2.98)	14.2 (2.02)
Q3	55.3 (2.49)	29.8 (2.59)	15.0 (1.94)
Q4	51.3 (3.29)	26.3 (4.20)	19.0 (3.26)
2009	53.2 (1.51)	29.4 (1.27)	17.4 (1.04)
Q1	53.0 (3.28)	28.3 (3.25)	17.7 (2.56)
Q2	52.5 (2.64)	29.0 (2.04)	18.7 (1.81)
Q3	53.5 (3.02)	30.2 (2.51)	16.5 (2.15)
Q4	53.8 (1.97)	29.9 (1.76)	16.6 (1.25)
2010	53.7 (1.32)	29.2 (1.14)	17.3 (0.98)
Q1	52.4 (2.86)	31.4 (2.62)	16.7 (1.71)
Q2	58.7 (2.44)	26.4 (1.84)	14.6 (1.74)
Q3	54.6 (2.14)	26.9 (1.73)	18.1 (1.76)
Q4	49.4 (2.72)	31.9 (2.37)	19.6 (1.89)
2011	47.1 (1.27)	34.0 (1.27)	19.2 (0.99)
Q1	48.2 (2.74)	33.9 (3.88)	18.1 (2.33)
Q2	46.3 (2.32)	34.8 (2.35)	19.1 (1.73)
Q3	47.7 (2.15)	33.2 (2.09)	19.8 (1.63)
Q4	46.4 (2.09)	34.6 (2.24)	19.3 (1.66)
2012	46.6 (1.67)	34.2 (1.50)	20.0 (1.16)
Q1	50.3 (2.98)	34.0 (2.80)	16.2 (1.64)
Q2	45.2 (2.47)	35.1 (2.51)	20.8 (1.93)
Q3	45.8 (2.92)	33.6 (2.56)	21.0 (2.54)
Q4	45.3 (2.96)	34.3 (2.64)	21.4 (2.15)
Non-Hispanic, white, single race			
2008	24.2 (0.99)	65.3 (1.23)	11.1 (0.74)
Q1	22.7 (1.90)	67.8 (2.20)	9.6 (1.13)
Q2	25.2 (1.60)	65.3 (1.85)	10.4 (1.16)
Q3	25.8 (1.71)	64.1 (1.99)	10.8 (1.18)
Q4	23.3 (2.54)	63.8 (3.06)	13.6 (1.98)
2009	25.5 (0.99)	63.0 (1.13)	11.9 (0.76)
Q1	22.2 (2.41)	67.6 (2.71)	10.6 (1.94)
Q2	27.2 (1.70)	61.6 (1.95)	11.4 (1.24)
Q3	27.6 (1.73)	60.5 (1.91)	12.3 (1.28)
Q4	25.3 (1.37)	62.0 (1.68)	13.6 (1.23)
2010	26.4 (0.87)	61.6 (1.07)	12.6 (0.68)
Q1	26.9 (1.72)	58.8 (2.13)	14.9 (1.42)
Q2	27.3 (1.65)	62.6 (1.95)	10.3 (1.06)
Q3	26.9 (1.84)	60.9 (2.17)	13.0 (1.41)
Q4	24.4 (1.57)	64.4 (1.94)	12.1 (1.31)
2011	20.4 (0.81)	67.1 (0.98)	13.4 (0.73)
Q1	23.5 (1.68)	63.0 (2.02)	14.0 (1.36)
Q2	19.8 (1.62)	69.7 (2.00)	11.0 (1.06)
Q3	21.4 (1.67)	65.1 (1.89)	14.6 (1.62)
Q4	16.7 (1.35)	70.8 (1.77)	13.7 (1.26)
2012	18.4 (0.83)	69.2 (0.97)	13.6 (0.69)
Q1	18.6 (1.66)	67.0 (2.05)	15.5 (1.45)
Q2	17.7 (1.68)	71.8 (2.11)	11.8 (1.08)
Q3	18.4 (1.44)	67.8 (1.99)	14.9 (1.54)
Q4	18.8 (1.38)	70.3 (1.76)	11.9 (1.12)

See footnotes at end of table.

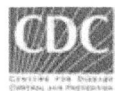

Table 11. Percentages of persons aged 19–25 who were uninsured, had private health insurance coverage, and had public health plan coverage at the time of interview, by race/ethnicity, year, and quarter: United States, January 2008–December 2012 (cont.)

Race/ethnicity, year, and quarter (Q)	Uninsured[1]	Private health insurance coverage[2]	Public health plan coverage[3]
		Percent (standard error)	
Non-Hispanic, black, single race			
2008	34.6 (2.21)	41.5 (1.71)	25.5 (2.70)
Q1	35.8 (4.76)	42.2 (3.00)	26.5 (7.24)
Q2	29.8 (2.76)	43.1 (3.61)	28.6 (3.26)
Q3	30.0 (2.60)	45.9 (3.01)	24.7 (2.39)
Q4	43.2 (4.81)	34.6 (4.46)	22.3 (3.88)
2009	38.0 (1.84)	36.6 (2.07)	25.4 (1.52)
Q1	38.3 (4.85)	38.1 (5.23)	23.4 (3.82)
Q2	39.2 (3.04)	38.1 (3.57)	22.9 (2.41)
Q3	41.0 (3.08)	32.6 (3.10)	26.4 (2.75)
Q4	33.8 (2.56)	37.7 (3.07)	28.7 (2.64)
2010	39.8 (1.70)	34.2 (1.72)	26.8 (1.42)
Q1	40.1 (2.92)	34.8 (2.83)	26.1 (2.99)
Q2	38.9 (3.10)	32.2 (2.98)	28.9 (2.71)
Q3	44.9 (3.04)	32.9 (3.09)	23.8 (2.62)
Q4	35.1 (3.16)	36.8 (3.42)	28.6 (2.96)
2011	33.0 (1.65)	41.5 (1.70)	27.0 (1.66)
Q1	35.8 (3.09)	39.0 (3.21)	25.9 (2.66)
Q2	32.4 (2.63)	43.9 (2.68)	26.6 (2.74)
Q3	31.0 (3.19)	41.0 (3.34)	28.5 (2.90)
Q4	32.3 (3.41)	43.1 (3.52)	26.3 (3.33)
2012	30.1 (1.52)	44.0 (1.47)	27.1 (1.56)
Q1	32.5 (2.72)	37.4 (2.97)	30.8 (3.10)
Q2	26.7 (2.43)	45.7 (3.63)	28.1 (3.03)
Q3	31.9 (2.87)	44.1 (3.12)	24.1 (2.62)
Q4	29.6 (3.45)	48.9 (3.37)	25.0 (2.91)

[1]A person was defined as uninsured if he or she did not have any private health insurance, Medicare, Medicaid, Children's Health Insurance Program (CHIP), state-sponsored or other government-sponsored health plan, or military plan. A person was also defined as uninsured if he or she had only Indian Health Service coverage or had only a private plan that paid for one type of service, such as accidents or dental care.
[2]Excludes plans that paid for only one type of service, such as accidents or dental care.
[3]Includes Medicaid, CHIP, state-sponsored or other government-sponsored health plan, Medicare (disability), and military plans.

NOTE: Data are based on household interviews of a sample of the civilian noninstitutionalized population.

DATA SOURCE: CDC/NCHS, National Health Interview Survey, 2008–2012, Family Core component.

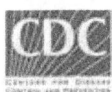

Table 12. Percentages of persons under age 65 with private coverage who were enrolled in a high-deductible health plan, in a high-deductible health plan without a health savings account, and in a consumer-directed health plan, and who were in a family with a flexible spending account for medical expenses, by year: United States, 2007–2012

Year	Enrolled in a high-deductible health plan (HDHP)[1]	Enrolled in an HDHP without a health savings account (HSA)[2]	Enrolled in a consumer-directed health Plan (CDHP)[3]	In a family with a flexible spending account (FSA) for medical expenses
	Percent (standard error)			
2007	17.5 (0.51)	12.9 (0.43)	4.5 (0.30)	16.7 (0.55)
2008	19.2 (0.55)	14.1 (0.46)	5.2 (0.29)	18.7 (0.58)
2009	22.5 (0.58)	15.9 (0.43)	6.6 (0.33)	20.4 (0.50)
2010	25.3 (0.54)	17.6 (0.46)	7.7 (0.33)	20.4 (0.50)
2011	29.0 (0.54)	19.9 (0.41)	9.2 (0.35)	21.4 (0.53)
2012	31.1 (0.57)	20.3 (0.42)	10.8 (0.34)	21.6 (0.45)

[1]A high-deductible health plan (HDHP) was defined in 2010 through 2012 as a health plan with an annual deductible of at least $1,200 for self-only coverage and $2,400 for family coverage. The deductible is adjusted annually for inflation. For 2009, the annual deductible for self-only coverage was $1,250 and for family coverage was $2,300. For 2007 and 2008, the annual deductible for self-only coverage was $1,100 and for family coverage was $2,200.
[2]A health savings account (HSA) is a tax-advantaged account or fund that can be used to pay for medical expenses. It must be coupled with an HDHP.
[3]A consumer-directed health plan (CDHP) is an HDHP coupled with an HSA.

NOTES: The measures of HDHP enrollment, CDHP enrollment, and being in a family with an FSA for medical expenses are not mutually exclusive. Therefore, a person may be counted in more than one measure. The individual components of HDHPs may not add up to the total, due to rounding. Data are based on household interviews of a sample of the civilian noninstitutionalized population.

DATA SOURCE: CDC/NCHS, National Health Interview Survey, 2007–2012, Family Core component.

Table 13. Percentages of persons under age 65 with private coverage who were enrolled in a high-deductible health plan, by year and source of private coverage: United States, 2007–2012

Year	Employment-based[1]	Directly purchased[2]
	Percent (standard error)	
2007	15.6 (0.53)	39.2 (1.82)
2008	17.1 (0.53)	44.7 (1.84)
2009	20.2 (0.59)	46.9 (1.84)
2010	23.3 (0.54)	48.0 (1.48)
2011	26.9 (0.53)	52.4 (1.49)
2012	29.2 (0.60)	54.7 (1.61)

[1]Private insurance that was originally obtained through a present or former employer or union or through a professional association.
[2]Private insurance that was originally obtained through direct purchase or through other means not related to employment.

NOTE: Data are based on household interviews of a sample of the civilian noninstitutionalized population.

DATA SOURCE: CDC/NCHS, National Health Interview Survey, 2007–2012, Family Core component.

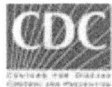

Table 14. Percentages of persons in selected states who lacked health insurance coverage, had public health plan coverage, or had private health insurance coverage at the time of interview, by age group: United States, 2012

Age group and state	Uninsured[1]	Public[2] health plan coverage	Private[3] health insurance coverage
		Percent (standard error)	
All ages[4]			
All states[5]	14.7 (0.21)	33.4 (0.31)	59.6 (0.39)
Alabama	12.9 (1.50)	34.7 (2.28)	63.1 (2.84)
Arizona	20.1 (1.70)	37.2 (2.19)	49.4 (2.78)
Arkansas	18.0 (1.74)	38.7 (2.35)	51.6 (2.97)
California	17.2 (0.50)	33.2 (0.86)	54.1 (1.08)
Colorado	11.7 (1.43)	29.3 (2.16)	63.6 (2.80)
Connecticut	9.6 (1.29)	31.4 (2.17)	67.6 (2.69)
Florida	19.8 (0.92)	37.6 (1.40)	49.1 (1.46)
Georgia	18.5 (1.40)	32.7 (1.25)	53.7 (1.63)
Hawaii	5.8 (1.26)	42.3 (2.83)	67.3 (3.31)
Idaho	18.4 (1.80)	33.8 (2.35)	57.9 (3.01)
Illinois	12.5 (0.85)	27.8 (1.39)	67.3 (1.66)
Indiana	13.0 (1.46)	34.0 (2.20)	64.0 (2.74)
Iowa	8.2 (1.25)	30.9 (2.24)	74.8 (2.58)
Kansas	12.9 (1.54)	29.0 (2.22)	66.9 (2.84)
Kentucky	14.8 (1.63)	39.6 (2.39)	54.4 (2.99)
Louisiana	13.7 (1.58)	38.1 (2.37)	54.9 (2.99)
Maine	7.6 (1.40)	34.9 (2.69)	65.3 (3.30)
Maryland	9.9 (1.29)	29.2 (2.09)	68.6 (2.62)
Massachusetts	4.8 (0.94)	34.2 (2.22)	71.7 (2.60)
Michigan	11.2 (1.14)	31.3 (1.32)	69.0 (1.91)
Minnesota	7.4 (1.18)	26.1 (2.11)	77.1 (2.48)
Mississippi	19.0 (1.74)	39.2 (2.31)	48.8 (2.91)
Missouri	15.2 (1.57)	33.4 (2.20)	59.2 (2.82)
Nebraska	13.5 (1.68)	28.9 (2.37)	69.0 (2.98)
Nevada	18.5 (1.70)	28.1 (2.09)	58.7 (2.82)
New Hampshire	13.6 (1.72)	32.6 (2.50)	65.3 (3.12)
New Jersey	11.3 (1.11)	27.1 (1.65)	69.9 (2.10)
New Mexico	16.6 (1.93)	51.1 (2.76)	40.6 (3.34)
New York	10.6 (0.70)	37.1 (1.26)	59.1 (1.43)
North Carolina	17.8 (1.62)	41.7 (1.38)	50.3 (2.88)
Ohio	11.8 (1.01)	32.3 (1.82)	63.8 (2.11)
Oklahoma	20.9 (1.90)	37.7 (2.41)	50.8 (3.06)
Oregon	15.9 (1.62)	30.8 (2.17)	62.8 (2.79)
Pennsylvania	11.2 (0.84)	31.8 (1.41)	66.2 (1.58)
Rhode Island	10.4 (1.63)	38.1 (2.76)	60.7 (3.41)
South Carolina	20.9 (1.86)	37.6 (2.36)	50.6 (2.99)
Tennessee	15.1 (1.63)	36.9 (2.34)	54.4 (2.97)
Texas	20.9 (0.85)	30.4 (1.23)	53.7 (1.57)
Utah	16.4 (1.47)	24.3 (1.81)	65.8 (2.46)
Virginia	11.7 (1.23)	32.5 (1.91)	65.3 (2.39)
Washington	16.2 (1.52)	31.7 (2.05)	60.6 (2.65)
West Virginia	15.1 (1.59)	42.7 (2.34)	52.5 (2.90)
Wisconsin	11.9 (1.44)	33.8 (2.24)	68.6 (2.70)

See footnotes at end of table.

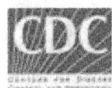

Table 14. Percentages of persons in selected states who lacked health insurance coverage, had public health plan coverage, or had private health insurance coverage at the time of interview, by age group: United States, 2012 (cont.)

Age group and state	Uninsured[1]	Public[2] health plan coverage	Private[3] health insurance coverage
		Percent (standard error)	
Under 65 years[4]			
All states[5]	16.9 (0.24)	23.5 (0.31)	61.0 (0.42)
Alabama	15.0 (1.74)	24.1 (2.27)	63.4 (3.08)
Arizona	23.6 (1.93)	26.4 (2.19)	51.0 (2.99)
Arkansas	21.7 (2.02)	26.4 (2.36)	53.5 (3.21)
California	19.3 (0.56)	24.9 (0.92)	56.4 (1.12)
Colorado	13.3 (1.59)	20.7 (2.08)	66.8 (2.91)
Connecticut	10.9 (1.46)	21.6 (2.10)	68.9 (2.84)
Florida	23.9 (1.12)	25.0 (0.99)	52.2 (1.58)
Georgia	20.5 (1.57)	24.9 (1.11)	55.8 (1.65)
Hawaii	7.6 (1.61)	26.2 (2.93)	68.2 (3.74)
Idaho	21.2 (2.04)	23.6 (2.32)	58.1 (3.24)
Illinois	14.1 (0.98)	18.4 (1.31)	68.1 (1.84)
Indiana	15.1 (1.68)	23.3 (2.16)	63.2 (2.97)
Iowa	9.7 (1.46)	18.3 (2.08)	73.7 (2.85)
Kansas	14.6 (1.71)	19.3 (2.09)	67.1 (3.00)
Kentucky	16.9 (1.84)	31.1 (2.49)	55.8 (3.21)
Louisiana	15.8 (1.79)	28.6 (2.42)	57.8 (3.18)
Maine	8.8 (1.62)	25.6 (2.72)	67.6 (3.51)
Maryland	11.2 (1.45)	20.1 (2.01)	69.5 (2.78)
Massachusetts	5.7 (1.11)	22.6 (2.18)	72.9 (2.79)
Michigan	12.8 (1.24)	21.0 (1.47)	68.7 (1.97)
Minnesota	8.4 (1.33)	15.9 (1.92)	78.0 (2.61)
Mississippi	22.0 (1.97)	30.1 (2.38)	49.4 (3.13)
Missouri	17.7 (1.79)	22.6 (2.15)	61.5 (3.01)
Nebraska	15.5 (1.91)	17.8 (2.21)	69.1 (3.21)
Nevada	21.0 (1.88)	18.3 (1.95)	62.5 (2.94)
New Hampshire	16.3 (2.02)	19.8 (2.38)	65.8 (3.41)
New Jersey	12.8 (1.24)	17.3 (1.53)	71.1 (2.20)
New Mexico	21.0 (2.33)	38.0 (3.04)	41.6 (3.71)
New York	12.0 (0.79)	28.1 (1.29)	61.1 (1.51)
North Carolina	21.5 (1.83)	29.8 (1.83)	50.1 (3.10)
Ohio	13.6 (1.12)	23.1 (1.86)	65.5 (2.35)
Oklahoma	24.2 (2.14)	28.0 (2.45)	50.1 (3.29)
Oregon	18.6 (1.87)	19.1 (2.06)	64.3 (3.02)
Pennsylvania	13.0 (0.94)	21.1 (1.27)	67.3 (1.69)
Rhode Island	12.1 (1.87)	27.6 (2.81)	62.2 (3.66)
South Carolina	25.1 (2.16)	25.1 (2.36)	51.2 (3.28)
Tennessee	17.4 (1.86)	26.8 (2.37)	56.6 (3.19)
Texas	23.2 (0.93)	22.4 (1.19)	55.3 (1.65)
Utah	17.8 (1.58)	18.4 (1.74)	66.1 (2.57)
Virginia	13.5 (1.40)	22.3 (1.86)	66.5 (2.53)
Washington	18.0 (1.68)	23.1 (2.01)	61.1 (2.80)
West Virginia	17.7 (1.84)	32.8 (2.47)	51.8 (3.16)
Wisconsin	14.1 (1.68)	21.3 (2.16)	67.4 (2.97)

See footnotes at end of table.

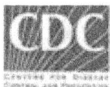

Table 14. Percentages of persons in selected states who lacked health insurance coverage, had public health plan coverage, or had private health insurance coverage at the time of interview, by age group: United States, 2012 (cont.)

Age group and state	Uninsured[1]	Public[2] health plan coverage	Private[3] health insurance coverage
		Percent (standard error)	
18–64 years[4]			
All states[5]	20.9 (0.29)	16.4 (0.25)	64.1 (0.39)
Alabama	18.5 (2.05)	17.0 (1.90)	67.5 (2.84)
Arizona	26.8 (1.33)	19.3 (1.93)	55.3 (2.93)
Arkansas	27.9 (2.52)	15.8 (1.90)	58.1 (3.09)
California	24.4 (0.68)	16.4 (0.78)	59.8 (1.08)
Colorado	16.7 (1.62)	16.4 (1.86)	67.5 (2.83)
Connecticut	13.6 (2.42)	16.4 (1.78)	71.4 (2.62)
Florida	28.9 (1.43)	16.3 (0.82)	55.9 (1.49)
Georgia	25.6 (1.83)	15.3 (1.16)	60.5 (1.82)
Hawaii	*9.5 (3.01)	19.6 (2.48)	72.9 (3.35)
Idaho	26.7 (2.49)	13.4 (1.84)	62.9 (3.15)
Illinois	18.3 (1.27)	11.5 (0.87)	71.0 (1.60)
Indiana	17.3 (2.41)	16.5 (1.85)	68.0 (2.80)
Iowa	13.0 (1.95)	12.5 (1.73)	76.1 (2.69)
Kansas	19.3 (2.61)	11.0 (1.67)	71.1 (2.92)
Kentucky	22.2 (2.31)	20.9 (2.11)	60.1 (3.06)
Louisiana	21.2 (2.56)	20.4 (2.10)	60.3 (3.06)
Maine	11.2 (1.88)	23.5 (2.50)	67.3 (3.33)
Maryland	12.4 (2.15)	14.8 (1.69)	73.6 (2.53)
Massachusetts	*6.6 (2.24)	20.1 (1.97)	74.4 (2.58)
Michigan	16.1 (1.56)	14.7 (1.23)	70.9 (2.05)
Minnesota	9.7 (2.09)	13.5 (1.74)	78.7 (2.51)
Mississippi	27.3 (1.82)	19.7 (1.98)	54.7 (2.98)
Missouri	22.0 (2.29)	17.0 (1.89)	62.6 (2.94)
Nebraska	17.1 (2.75)	10.5 (1.73)	73.9 (2.98)
Nevada	24.7 (2.25)	14.5 (1.75)	62.9 (2.89)
New Hampshire	20.5 (1.96)	13.9 (1.97)	67.6 (3.21)
New Jersey	16.4 (1.91)	12.1 (1.29)	72.8 (2.11)
New Mexico	27.5 (2.89)	25.0 (2.66)	48.3 (3.70)
New York	14.7 (0.90)	23.7 (1.15)	62.9 (1.48)
North Carolina	27.1 (2.35)	19.4 (1.63)	55.0 (3.10)
Ohio	16.6 (1.29)	17.4 (1.67)	67.9 (2.09)
Oklahoma	30.9 (2.41)	17.2 (1.99)	54.1 (3.17)
Oregon	22.7 (2.27)	13.5 (1.71)	65.4 (2.86)
Pennsylvania	15.9 (1.07)	15.0 (1.17)	70.5 (1.74)
Rhode Island	15.6 (2.67)	21.0 (2.47)	64.8 (3.49)
South Carolina	28.6 (2.18)	19.6 (2.04)	53.5 (3.09)
Tennessee	22.3 (2.13)	18.1 (1.99)	60.4 (3.04)
Texas	28.6 (1.13)	13.2 (0.85)	59.1 (1.45)
Utah	22.1 (2.01)	10.6 (1.44)	68.9 (2.61)
Virginia	16.8 (1.74)	17.6 (1.64)	68.1 (2.42)
Washington	22.6 (1.89)	13.9 (1.61)	65.5 (2.65)
West Virginia	23.2 (2.06)	26.3 (2.21)	52.7 (3.02)
Wisconsin	17.1 (1.84)	16.4 (1.89)	68.9 (2.85)

See footnotes at end of table.

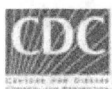

Table 14. Percentages of persons in selected states who lacked health insurance coverage, had public health plan coverage, or had private health insurance coverage at the time of interview, by age group: United States, 2012 (cont.)

Age group and state	Uninsured[1]	Public[2] health plan coverage	Private[3] health insurance coverage
		Percent (standard error)	
0–17 years[4]			
All states[5]	6.6 (0.26)	42.1 (0.62)	52.8 (0.63)
Alabama	*4.6 (1.74)	45.1 (5.07)	51.2 (4.90)
Arizona	15.6 (2.59)	44.1 (4.34)	40.2 (4.12)
Arkansas	*5.6 (1.83)	53.4 (4.86)	41.8 (4.63)
California	6.7 (0.58)	46.2 (1.58)	47.8 (1.55)
Colorado	*4.3 (1.53)	31.6 (4.26)	65.1 (4.21)
Connecticut	†	38.8 (4.88)	60.5 (4.71)
Florida	9.6 (1.43)	49.4 (2.69)	41.7 (2.40)
Georgia	8.4 (1.70)	48.0 (3.03)	44.5 (2.42)
Idaho	8.9 (2.19)	46.7 (4.71)	47.3 (4.53)
Illinois	2.7 (0.66)	37.3 (2.92)	60.1 (3.00)
Indiana	9.2 (2.18)	41.0 (4.55)	50.6 (4.45)
Iowa	†	33.1 (4.59)	67.5 (4.40)
Kansas	*5.1 (1.60)	36.3 (4.29)	58.9 (4.22)
Kentucky	*2.9 (1.35)	57.8 (4.89)	44.7 (4.74)
Louisiana	*2.8 (1.33)	48.2 (4.88)	51.6 (4.69)
Maryland	7.5 (2.08)	36.1 (4.65)	57.3 (4.61)
Massachusetts	†	31.3 (4.78)	67.9 (4.63)
Michigan	5.0 (1.21)	36.0 (2.93)	63.4 (2.64)
Minnesota	*5.1 (1.71)	22.7 (3.99)	76.3 (3.90)
Mississippi	7.3 (2.08)	59.1 (4.83)	34.6 (4.50)
Missouri	7.6 (1.97)	35.5 (4.37)	59.0 (4.33)
Nebraska	11.5 (2.69)	35.7 (4.96)	57.2 (4.93)
Nevada	12.2 (2.37)	27.4 (3.95)	61.6 (4.14)
New Jersey	3.9 (1.16)	30.4 (3.35)	66.7 (3.30)
New York	3.5 (0.78)	41.6 (2.51)	55.5 (2.45)
North Carolina	8.2 (1.41)	55.1 (3.59)	38.3 (3.60)
Ohio	5.6 (1.24)	37.8 (3.04)	59.3 (3.47)
Oklahoma	*6.9 (2.08)	55.9 (4.99)	39.6 (4.73)
Oregon	*6.1 (1.95)	36.5 (4.79)	60.6 (4.68)
Pennsylvania	4.2 (1.11)	39.2 (3.32)	57.8 (3.08)
South Carolina	13.8 (3.01)	42.7 (5.29)	44.0 (5.11)
Tennessee	*4.0 (1.59)	50.5 (4.95)	46.1 (4.74)
Texas	11.0 (1.18)	42.8 (2.42)	46.7 (2.36)
Utah	10.7 (1.81)	30.9 (3.32)	61.7 (3.36)
Virginia	*4.5 (1.39)	35.3 (3.93)	62.2 (3.84)
Washington	*5.2 (1.59)	48.6 (4.36)	48.7 (4.20)
West Virginia	*2.9 (1.37)	50.2 (4.99)	49.3 (4.80)
Wisconsin	*5.9 (1.85)	34.7 (4.56)	63.3 (4.44)

* Estimate has a relative standard error (RSE) greater than 30% and less than or equal to 50% and should be used with caution as it does not meet standards of reliability or precision.
† Estimate has an RSE greater than 50% and is not shown.
[1]A person was defined as uninsured if he or she did not have any private health insurance, Medicare, Medicaid, Children's Health Insurance Program (CHIP), state-sponsored or other government-sponsored health plan, or military plan. A person was also defined as uninsured if he or she had only Indian Health Service coverage or had only a private plan that paid for one type of service, such as accidents or dental care.
[2]Includes Medicaid, Children's Health Insurance Program (CHIP), state-sponsored or other government-sponsored health plan, Medicare (disability), and military plans.
[3]Excludes plans that paid for only one type of service, such as accidents or dental care. A small number of persons were covered by both public and private plans and were included in both categories.
[4]Estimates are presented for fewer than 50 states and the District of Columbia due to considerations of sample size and precision.
[5]Includes all 50 states and the District of Columbia.

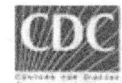

NOTE: Data are based on household interviews of a sample of the civilian noninstitutionalized population.

DATA SOURCE: CDC/NCHS, National Health Interview Survey, 2012, Family Core component.

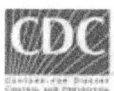

Technical Notes

The Centers for Disease Control and Prevention's (CDC) National Center for Health Statistics (NCHS) is releasing selected estimates of health insurance coverage for the civilian noninstitutionalized U.S. population based on data from the 2012 National Health Interview Survey (NHIS), along with comparable estimates from the 1997–2011 NHIS.

Three measures of lack of health insurance coverage are provided: (a) uninsured at the time of interview, (b) uninsured at least part of the year prior to interview (which also includes persons uninsured for more than a year), and (c) uninsured for more than a year at the time of interview. To reflect different policy-relevant perspectives, different time frames are used to measure lack of insurance coverage. The measure of uninsured at the time of interview provides an estimate of persons who at any given time may have experienced barriers to obtaining needed health care. The estimate of persons who were uninsured at any time in the year prior to interview provides an annual caseload of persons who may experience these barriers. This measure includes persons who have insurance at the time of interview but who had a period of noncoverage in the year prior to interview, as well as those who are currently uninsured and who may have been uninsured for a long period of time. Finally, the measure of lack of coverage for more than a year provides an estimate of those with a persistent lack of coverage who may be at high risk of not obtaining preventive services or care for illness and injury. These three measures of lack of coverage are not mutually exclusive, and a given individual may be counted in more than one of the measures. Estimates of enrollment in public and private coverage are also provided.

This report also includes estimates of three types of consumer-directed private health care. Consumer-directed health care may enable individuals to have more control over when and how they access care, what types of care they use, and how much they spend on health care services.

National attention to consumer-directed health care increased following enactment of the Medicare Prescription Drug Improvement and Modernization Act of 2003 (P.L. 108–173), which established tax-advantaged health savings accounts (HSAs) (1). In 2007, three additional questions were added to the health insurance section of NHIS to monitor enrollment in consumer-directed health care among persons with private health insurance. Estimates for 2012 are provided for enrollment in high-deductible health plans (HDHPs), plans with high deductibles coupled with HSAs (i.e., consumer-directed health plans; CDHPs), and being in a family with a flexible spending account (FSA) for medical expenses not otherwise covered. For a more complete description of consumer-directed health care, see "Definitions of selected terms" below.

The 2012 health insurance estimates are being released prior to final data editing and final weighting, to provide access to the most recent information from NHIS. Differences between estimates calculated using preliminary data files and final data files are typically less than 0.1 percentage point. However, preliminary estimates of persons without health insurance coverage are generally 0.1–0.3 percentage points lower than the final estimates due to the editing procedures used for the final data files.

Estimates for 2012 are stratified by age group, sex, race/ethnicity, poverty status, marital status, employment status, region, and educational attainment.

Data source

NHIS is a multistage probability sample survey of the civilian noninstitutionalized population of the United States and is the source of data for this report. The survey is conducted continuously throughout the year for NCHS by interviewers from the U.S. Census Bureau.

NHIS is a comprehensive health survey that can be used to relate health insurance coverage to health outcomes

and health care utilization. It has a low item nonresponse rate (about 1%) for the health insurance questions. Because NHIS is conducted throughout the year—yielding a nationally representative sample each month—data can be analyzed monthly or quarterly to monitor health insurance coverage trends.

The sample for NHIS is redesigned about every 10 years. A new sample design for NHIS was implemented in 2006. The fundamental structure of the current NHIS sample design is very similar to the previous 1995–2005 NHIS sample design. Oversampling of black and Hispanic populations has been retained, and the current sample design also oversamples the Asian population. The impact of the 2006 sample design on estimates presented in this report is minimal. Visit the NCHS website at: http://www.cdc.gov/nchs/nhis.htm for more information on the design, content, and use of NHIS.

The data for this report are derived from the Family Core component of the 1997–2012 NHIS, which collects information on all family members in each household. Data analyses for the 2012 NHIS were based on 108,131 persons in the Family Core.

Estimation procedures

NCHS creates survey weights for each calendar quarter of the NHIS sample. The NHIS data weighting procedure is described in more detail at: http://www.cdc.gov/nchs/data/series/sr_02/sr02_130.pdf. Estimates were calculated using NHIS survey weights, which are calibrated to census totals for sex, age, and race/ethnicity of the U.S. civilian noninstitutionalized population. The weights for 1997–1999 NHIS data were derived from 1990-census-based population estimates. Weights for 2000–2011 were derived from 2000-census-based population estimates. Beginning with the 2012 NHIS data, weights were derived from 2010-census-based population estimates.

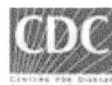

An error was made in the poststratification component of weights from January 2004 through 2008 for the preliminary estimates used in this report. The error affected "nonminority" person weights. Compared with the corrected weight estimates, those made with the original weights generally differ by 0.01 percentage point, and variances generally differ by 0.001 percentage point.

Point estimates, and estimates of their variances, were calculated using SUDAAN software to account for the complex sample design of NHIS, taking into account stratum and primary sampling unit (PSU) identifiers. The Taylor series linearization method was chosen for variance estimation.

The two Early Release (ER) reports released in June 2007 used final in-house design variables (stratum and PSU identifiers) for estimating variance for the 2006 estimates. ER reports other than the June 2007 update use ER interim design variables to estimate variance, with the exception of the state-level estimates, which use the final in-house design variables to estimate variance.

State-specific health insurance estimates are presented for 43 states for persons of all ages, persons under age 65, and adults aged 18–64. State-specific estimates are presented for 38 states for children aged 0–17. Estimates are not presented for all 50 states and the District of Columbia due to considerations of sample size and precision. States with fewer than 1,000 interviews for persons of all ages are excluded. In addition, estimates for children in states that did not have at least 300 children with completed interviews are not presented.

For the 10 states with the largest populations (California, Florida, Georgia, Illinois, Michigan, New York, North Carolina, Ohio, Pennsylvania, and Texas), standard errors (SEs) were calculated using SUDAAN. Because of small sample sizes and limitations in the NHIS design, similarly estimated SEs for other states could be statistically unstable or negatively biased;

consequently, for states other than the largest 10 states, an estimated design effect was used to calculate SEs. For this report, the design effect, *deff*, of a percentage is the ratio of the sampling variance of the percentage (taking into account the complex NHIS sample design) to the sampling variance of the percentage from a simple random sample (SRS) based on the same observed number of persons.

Therefore, for each health insurance measure and domain, SEs for the smaller states were calculated by multiplying the SRS SE by *A*, where *A* is the average value of the square root of *deff* over the 10 most populous states. Values of *A* ranged from 1.54 for uninsured children aged 0–17 years to 2.29 for persons of all ages with private coverage and 2.29 for persons under age 65 with private coverage.

Calculation of SE s of the differences between state and national estimates accounted for correlations.

Trends in coverage were assessed using Joinpoint regression (2), which characterizes trends as joined linear segments. A joinpoint is the year where two segments with different slopes meet. Joinpoint software uses statistical criteria to determine the fewest number of segments necessary to characterize a trend and the year(s) when segments begin and end.

Unless otherwise noted, all estimates shown meet the NCHS standard of having less than or equal to 30% relative standard error. Differences between percentages or rates were evaluated using two-sided significance tests at the 0.05 level. Terms such as "greater than" and "less than" indicate a statistically significant difference. Terms such as "similar" and "no difference" indicate that the estimates being compared were not significantly different. Lack of comment regarding the difference between any two estimates does not necessarily mean that the difference was tested and found to be not significant.

Definitions of selected terms

Health insurance coverage—
The "Private health insurance coverage" category includes persons who had any comprehensive private insurance plan (including health maintenance and preferred provider organizations). These plans include those obtained through an employer, purchased directly, or purchased through local or community programs. Private coverage excludes plans that pay for only one type of service, such as accidents or dental care. The "Public health plan coverage" category includes Medicaid, Children's Health Insurance Program (CHIP), state-sponsored or other government-sponsored health plans, Medicare, and military plans. A small number of persons were covered by both public and private plans and were included in both categories. A person was defined as uninsured if he or she did not have any private health insurance, Medicare, Medicaid, CHIP, state-sponsored or other government-sponsored health plan, or military plan, at the time of interview. A person was also defined as uninsured if he or she had only Indian Health Service coverage or had only a private plan that paid for one type of service, such as accidents or dental care. The analyses excluded persons with unknown health insurance status (about 1% of respondents each year).

Data on health insurance status were edited using an automated system based on logic checks and keyword searches. Information from follow-up questions, such as plan name(s), was used to reassign insurance status and type of coverage to avoid misclassification. For comparability, the estimates for all years were created using these same procedures.

The terms HIKIND, MCAREPRB, and MCAIDPRB refer to questions in NHIS. Data on type of health insurance are collected through the HIKIND question: *What kind of health insurance or health care coverage [do you/does person's name] have? INCLUDE those that pay for only one type of service (nursing home care, accidents, or dental care). EXCLUDE private plans that only provide extra cash while hospitalized.*

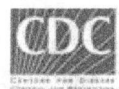

Respondents can indicate private and public plans or indicate that they or family members are not covered by insurance.

Two additional questions were added to the health insurance section of NHIS beginning with the third quarter of 2004. One question, MCAREPRB, was asked of persons aged 65 and over who had not indicated that they had Medicare. The MCAREPRB question is: *People covered by Medicare have a card which looks like this. [Are you/Is person's name] covered by Medicare?* The other question, MCAIDPRB, was asked of persons under age 65 who had not indicated any type of coverage. The MCAIDPRB question is: *There is a program called Medicaid that pays for health care for persons in need. In this State it is also called [state name]. [Are you/Is person's name] covered by Medicaid?*

Respondents who were considered insured at the time of interview were asked about periods of noncoverage in the past year. For persons who did not have health insurance at the time of interview, a question was asked concerning the length of time since the respondent had coverage. Respondents who originally classified themselves as uninsured but whose classification was changed to Medicare or Medicaid on the basis of a "yes" response to either probe question subsequently received appropriate follow-up questions concerning periods of noncoverage for insured respondents.

Method 1 estimates are based solely on responses to one question (HIKIND). Method 2 estimates are based on responses to three questions (HIKIND, MCAREPRB, and MCAIDPRB). Prior to 2004, estimates in earlier releases of this report were generated using Method 1. Estimates for 2004 are presented using Method 2 in the figures and both Method 1 and Method 2 in the tables. Estimates using Method 1 for the "Uninsured for more than a year" measure excluded persons whose classification was changed from "Uninsured" to either Medicare or Medicaid coverage by either additional probe question. As a result, these

respondents did not receive the follow-up question concerning how long it had been since they had coverage. However, they were asked the questions concerning noncoverage in the past 12 months for insured persons. Beginning in 2005, all estimates are calculated using all three questions (Method 2).

Of the 892 people (unweighted) who were eligible to receive the MCAREPRB question in the third and fourth quarters of 2004, 55.4% indicated they were covered by Medicare. Of the 9,146 people (unweighted) who were eligible to receive the MCAIDPRB question in the third and fourth quarters of 2004, 3.0% indicated they were covered by Medicaid.

From July through December 2004 (the third and fourth quarters combined), the estimates (weighted) for the "Uninsured at the time of interview" measure decreased from 10.4% to 9.9% for children under age 18, from 19.7% to 19.5% for adults aged 18–64, and from 1.7% to 1.2% for persons aged 65 and over with the use of Method 2 as compared with Method 1. The estimates for public coverage increased from 28.1% to 29.6% for children under age 18, from 11.3% to 11.4% for adults aged 18–64, and from 89.5% to 93.3% for persons aged 65 and over with the use of Method 2 as compared with Method 1. The tabulation of "Uninsured for more than a year" using Method 1 excludes respondents whose classification was changed to Medicare or Medicaid by either probe question because these individuals did not receive the question concerning duration of noncoverage for persons who are uninsured. The two additional questions had no impact on the estimates for private coverage. Additional information on the impact of these two probe questions on health insurance estimates can be found in "Impact of Medicare and Medicaid Probe Questions on Health Insurance Estimates From the National Health Interview Survey, 2004" (3).

Directly purchased coverage— Private insurance that was originally obtained through direct purchase or

through other means not related to employment.

Employment-based coverage— Private insurance that was originally obtained through a present or former employer or union or a professional association.

For persons with private health insurance, a new question regarding the annual deductible of each private health insurance plan was added beginning in 2007. For plans considered to be HDHPs, a follow-up question was asked regarding special accounts or funds used to pay for medical expenses: an HSA or a health reimbursement account (HRA). Lastly, a new question was added about family enrollment in an FSA for medical expenses.

High-deductible health plan (HDHP)—An HDHP was defined in 2010, 2011, and 2012 as a private health plan with an annual deductible of at least $1,200 for self-only coverage or $2,400 for family coverage. The deductible is adjusted annually for inflation. For 2009, the annual deductible for self-only coverage was $1,150 and for family coverage was $2,300. For 2007 and 2008, the annual deductible for self-only coverage was $1,100 and for family coverage was $2,200.

Consumer-directed health plan (CDHP)—A CDHP is defined as an HDHP with a special account to pay for medical expenses. Unspent funds are carried over to subsequent years. A person is considered to have a CDHP if there was a "yes" response to the following question: *With this plan, is there a special account or fund that can be used to pay for medical expenses? The accounts are sometimes referred to as Health Savings Accounts (HSAs), Health Reimbursement Accounts (HRAs), Personal Care accounts, Personal Medical funds, or Choice funds, and are different from Flexible Spending Accounts.*

Health savings account (HSA)— An HSA is a tax-advantaged account or fund that can be used to pay for medical expenses. It must be coupled with an HDHP. The funds contributed to the account are not subject to federal income tax at the time of deposit.

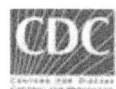

Unlike with FSAs, HSA funds roll over and accumulate year to year if not spent. HSAs are owned by the individual. Funds may be used to pay for qualified medical expenses at any time without federal tax liability. HSAs may also be referred to as Health Reimbursement Accounts (HRAs), Personal Care accounts, Personal Medical funds, or Choice funds, and the term "HSA" in this report includes accounts that use these alternative names.

Flexible spending account (FSA) for medical expenses—A person is considered to be in a family with an FSA if there was a "yes" response to the following question: *[Do you/Does anyone in your family] have a Flexible Spending Account for health expenses? These accounts are offered by some employers to allow employees to set aside pre-tax dollars of their own money for their use throughout the year to reimburse themselves for their out-of-pocket expenses for health care. With this type of account, any money remaining in the account at the end of the year, following a short grace period, is lost to the employee.*

The measures of HDHP enrollment, CDHP enrollment, and being in a family with an FSA for medical expenses are not mutually exclusive. Therefore, a person may be counted in more than one measure.

Education—The categories of education are based on the years of school completed or highest degree obtained for persons aged 18 and over. Only years completed in a school that advances a person toward an elementary or high school diploma, a General Educational Development high school equivalency diploma (GED), or a college, university, or professional degree are included. Education in other schools, or home schooling, is counted only if the credits are accepted in a regular school system.

Employment—Employment status is assessed at the time of interview and is obtained for persons aged 18 and over. In this release, it is presented only for persons aged 18–64.

Hispanic or Latino origin and race—Hispanic or Latino origin and race are two separate and distinct categories. Persons of Hispanic or Latino origin may be of any race. Hispanic or Latino origin includes persons of Mexican, Puerto Rican, Cuban, Central and South American, or Spanish origin. Race is based on the family respondent's description of his or her own race background, as well as the race background of other family members. For conciseness, the text, tables, and figures in this report use shorter versions of the 1997 Office of Management and Budget (OMB) terms for race and Hispanic or Latino origin. For example, the category "Not Hispanic or Latino, black or African American, single race" is referred to as "non-Hispanic black, single race" in the text, tables, and figures. Estimates for non-Hispanic persons of races other than white only, black only, and Asian only, or of multiple races, are combined into the "Other races or multiple race" category.

Poverty status—Poverty categories are based on the ratio of the family's income in the previous calendar year to the appropriate poverty threshold (given the family's size and number of children) defined by the U.S. Census Bureau for that year (4–19). Persons categorized as "Poor" have a ratio less than 1.0 (i.e., their family income was below the poverty threshold); "Near-poor" persons have incomes of 100% to less than 200% of the poverty threshold; and "Not-poor" persons have incomes that are 200% of the poverty threshold or greater. The remaining group of respondents is coded as "Unknown" with respect to poverty status. The percentage of respondents with unknown poverty status (19.1% in 1997, 23.6% in 1998, 26.4% in 1999, 27.0% in 2000, 27.1% in 2001, 28.1% in 2002, 31.5% in 2003, 29.6% in 2004, 28.9% in 2005, 30.7% in 2006, 18.0% in 2007, 15.8% in 2008, 12.3% in 2009, 12.2% in 2010, 11.5% in 2011 and 11.4% in 2012) is disaggregated by insurance status and age in Tables 4, 5, and 6.

In 2004, the NHIS instrument recorded a much larger than expected proportion of respondents with a family income for the previous calendar year of "$2." The ER updates from March 2005 through December 2005 used these preliminary data. Following extensive review, the "$2" responses were coded to "Not ascertained" for the final 2004 NHIS microdata files. The 2004 estimates of coverage by poverty status were recalculated using the final microdata. The revised estimates were released in the March 2006 ER update and continue to be used in subsequent ER updates. The problem with the "$2" income reports was fixed in the 2005 NHIS.

For more information on unknown income and unknown poverty status, see the *NHIS Survey Description* document for years 1997–2011 (available from: http://www.cdc.gov/nchs/nhis htm).

Prior to 2007, the "Income and Assets" section in the Family Core component of the NHIS instrument allowed respondents to report their family income in several ways. Respondents were first asked to provide their combined family income before taxes from all sources for the previous calendar year in a dollar amount (from $0 to $999,995). Respondents who did not know or refused to state an amount were then asked if their combined family income in the previous calendar year was $20,000 or more, or less than $20,000. If they again refused to answer or said they did not know, they were not asked any more questions about their family income. Respondents who did reply to the above-below-$20,000 question were then handed a list (flash card) of detailed income categories (top-coded at "$75,000 or more") and asked to select the interval containing their best estimate of their combined family income. Thus, NHIS respondents fell into one of four categories with respect to combined family income information: (a) those willing to supply a dollar amount; (b) those who indicated their combined family income from a fairly detailed set of intervals; (c) those who said that their combined family income was either $20,000 or more, or less than $20,000;

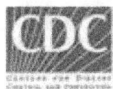

and (d) those unwilling to provide any information whatsoever. However, the flash card approach had a very low item response rate (15%–18%), and this led to income variables such as poverty ratio having relatively high levels of missing data (approximately 30% item nonresponse rate).

In the 2007 NHIS, the family income section of the questionnaire was redesigned to improve the collection of income information and reduce the amount of income nonresponse. Questions used to collect income data from respondents who initially would not indicate the amount of their family's income in the last calendar year were changed from using a flash card approach to using a set of unfolding brackets. The unfolding bracket method asks a series of closed-ended income range questions (e.g., "Is it less than $50,000?") if the respondent did not provide an answer to an exact income amount question. These questions utilize a series of income intervals, and respondents answering the complete path of questions would answer either two or three questions. The first follow-up income question asks a respondent if the family's income is less than $50,000. With this as a starting point, for respondents who answer "yes" to this question, additional questions are asked to determine if the family's income is below $35,000 and if the family's income is below the poverty threshold. Alternately, for respondents who answer "no" to the less-than-$50,000 question, additional questions are asked to determine if the family income is below $100,000 and below $75,000. The pilot test used to develop these questions is described elsewhere (20).

Based on preliminary data from the first quarter of 2007, 56% of the respondents eligible for the modified income follow-up questions answered all the questions in the applicable path. Initial evaluations of the distribution of poverty among selected demographic variables in the first quarter of 2007 suggest that poverty estimates are generally comparable with years 2006 and earlier (21). As a result of the changes in the questions, the 2007

through 2010 poverty ratio variable has fewer missing values compared with prior years. This reflects improved income item response rates.

In 2011, several new unfolding-bracket income questions were added to NHIS to improve the assignment of poverty status. Additional questions focused on assessing whether a family's income was less than 200% of the poverty threshold or 200% of the poverty threshold or more. The question received was dependent on family size. In addition, a question was added for respondents who answered that their family's income was $100,000 or more as to whether their family's income was less than $150,000, or $150,000 or more.

NCHS imputes income for approximately 30% of NHIS records. Beginning with survey year 2007, the imputation procedure was modified to take into account the changes made to the income section. The imputed income files are released a few months after the annual release of NHIS microdata and are not available for the ER updates. Therefore, ER health insurance estimates stratified by poverty status are based on reported income only and may differ from similar estimates produced later [e.g., in *Health, United States* (22)] that are based on both reported and imputed income.

Region—In the geographic classification of the U.S. population, states are grouped into the following four regions used by the U.S. Census Bureau:

Region   States included

Northeast Maine, Vermont, New Hampshire, Massachusetts, Connecticut, Rhode Island, New York, New Jersey, and Pennsylvania

Midwest Ohio, Illinois, Indiana, Michigan, Wisconsin, Minnesota, Iowa, Missouri, North Dakota, South Dakota, Kansas, and Nebraska

South Delaware, Maryland, District of Columbia,

West Virginia, Virginia, Kentucky, Tennessee, North Carolina, South Carolina, Georgia, Florida, Alabama, Mississippi, Louisiana, Oklahoma, Arkansas, and Texas

West Washington, Oregon, California, Nevada, New Mexico, Arizona, Idaho, Utah, Colorado, Montana, Wyoming, Alaska, and Hawaii

Additional Early Release Program Products

Two additional periodical reports are published through the ER Program. *Early Release of Selected Estimates Based on Data From the National Health Interview Survey* (23) is published quarterly and provides estimates of 15 selected measures of health, including insurance coverage. Other measures of health include estimates of having a usual place to go for medical care, obtaining needed medical care, influenza vaccination, pneumococcal vaccination, obesity, leisure-time physical activity, current smoking, alcohol consumption, HIV testing, general health status, personal care needs, serious psychological distress, diagnosed diabetes, and asthma episodes and current asthma.

Wireless Substitution: Early Release of Estimates From the National Health Interview Survey (24) is published in June and December and provides selected estimates of telephone coverage in the United States.

Other ER reports and tabulations on special topics are released on an as-needed basis. See: http://www.cdc.gov/nchs/nhis/releases. htm.

In addition to these reports, preliminary microdata files containing selected NHIS variables are produced as part of the ER Program. For each data collection year (January through December), these variables are made available three times: in about September (with data from the first

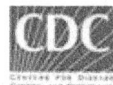

quarter), in about December (with data from the first two quarters), and in about March of the next year (with data from the first three quarters). NHIS data users can analyze these files through the NCHS Research Data Center without having to wait for the final annual NHIS microdata files to be released.

New measures and products may be added as work continues and in response to changing data needs. Feedback on these releases is welcome (e-mail).

Announcements about ERs, other new data releases, publications, and corrections related to NHIS will be sent to members of the HISUSERS electronic mailing list. To join, visit the CDC website at: http://www.cdc.gov/subscribe.html.

Suggested citation

Cohen RA, Martinez ME. Health insurance coverage: Early release of estimates from the National Health Interview Survey, 2012. National Center for Health Statistics. June 2013. Available from: http://www.cdc.gov/nchs/nhis/releases.htm.